AOSpine Masters Series

Spinal Infections

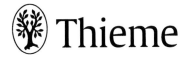

AOSpine Masters Series

Spinal Infections

Series Editor:
Luiz Roberto Vialle, MD, PhD
Professor of Orthopedics, School of Medicine
Catholic University of Parana State
Spine Unit
Curitiba, Brazil

Guest Editors:
S. Rajasekaran, MS ORTHO, FRCS, FACS, MCh ORTHO, PhD
Director and Chairman
Department of Orthopaedics & Spine Surgery
Ganga Hospital
Coimbatore, India

Rishi M. Kanna, MS, MRCS, FNB SPINE
Consultant Spine Surgeon
Ganga Hospital
Coimbatore, India

Giuseppe Barbagallo, MD
Department of Neurosciences
University of Catania
Catania, Italy

With 86 figures

Thieme
New York • Stuttgart • Delhi • Rio de Janeiro

Thieme Medical Publishers, Inc.
333 Seventh Ave.
New York, NY 10001

Executive Editor: William Lamsback
Managing Editor: Sarah Landis
Director, Editorial Services: Mary Jo Casey
Editorial Assistant: Haley Paskalides
Production Editor: Barbara A. Chernow
International Production Director: Andreas Schabert
Editorial Director: Sue Hodgson
International Marketing Director: Fiona Henderson
International Sales Director: Louisa Turrell
Director of Institutional Sales: Adam Bernacki
Senior Vice President and Chief Operating Officer: Sarah Vanderbilt
President: Brian D. Scanlan
Compositor: Carol Pierson, Chernow Editorial Services, Inc.

Library of Congress Cataloging-in-Publication Data
Names: Vialle, Luiz Roberto, editor. | Rajasekaran, S., editor. | Kanna, Rishi M., editor. | Barbagallo, Giuseppe, 1951– editor. | AOspine International (Firm)
Title: AOspine masters series. V. 10, Spinal infections / guest editors: Luiz Roberto Vialle, Shanmuganathan Rajasekaran, Rishi M. Kanna, Giuseppe Barbagallo.
Other titles: Spinal infections
Description: New York : Thieme, [2018] | Includes bibliographical references and index. |
Identifiers: LCCN 2018011119 (print) | LCCN 2018011922 (ebook) | ISBN 9781626234567 | ISBN 9781626234550 (alk. paper) | ISBN 9781626234567 (eISBN)
Subjects: | MESH: Spinal Diseases | Bacterial Infections | Spinal Cord Diseases | Bone Diseases, Infectious
Classification: LCC RD768 (ebook) | LCC RD768 (print) | NLM WE 727 | DDC 617.4/71--dc23
LC record available at https://lccn.loc.gov/2018011119

Important note: Medicine is an ever-changing science undergoing continual development. Research and clinical experience are continually expanding our knowledge, in particular our knowledge of proper treatment and drug therapy. Insofar as this book mentions any dosage or application, readers may rest assured that the authors, editors, and publishers have made every effort to ensure that such references are in accordance with the **state of knowledge at the time of production of the book.**

Nevertheless, this does not involve, imply, or express any guarantee or responsibility on the part of the publishers in respect to any dosage instructions and forms of applications stated in the book. **Every user is requested to examine carefully** the manufacturers' leaflets accompanying each drug and to check, if necessary in consultation with a physician or specialist, whether the dosage schedules mentioned therein or the contraindications stated by the manufacturers differ from the statements made in the present book. Such examination is particularly important with drugs that are either rarely used or have been newly released on the market. Every dosage schedule or every form of application used is entirely at the user's own risk and responsibility. The authors and publishers request every user to report to the publishers any discrepancies or inaccuracies noticed. If errors in this work are found after publication, errata will be posted at www.thieme.com on the product description page.

Some of the product names, patents, and registered designs referred to in this book are in fact registered trademarks or proprietary names even though specific reference to this fact is not always made in the text. Therefore, the appearance of a name without designation as proprietary is not to be construed as a representation by the publisher that it is in the public domain.

Printed in the United States of America by King Printing
5 4 3 2 1
ISBN 978-1-62623-455-0

Also available as an e-book:
eISBN 978-1-62623-456-7

FSC
www.fsc.org
100%
Paper from well-managed forests
FSC® C103101

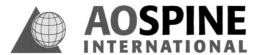

AOSpine Masters Series

Luiz Roberto Vialle, MD, PhD
Series Editor

Contents

Series Preface

Spine care is advancing at a rapid pace. The challenge for today's spine care professional is to quickly synthesize the best available evidence and expert opinion in the management of spine pathologies. The AOSpine Masters Series provides just that—each volume in the series delivers pathology-focused expert opinion on procedures, diagnosis, clinical wisdom, and pitfalls, and highlights today's top research papers.

To bring the value of its masters level educational courses and academic congresses to a wider audience, AOSpine has assembled internationally recognized spine pathology leaders to develop volumes in this Masters Series as a vehicle for sharing their experiences and expertise and providing links to the literature. Each volume focuses on a current compelling and sometimes controversial topic in spine care.

The unique and efficient format of the Masters Series volumes quickly focuses the attention of the reader on the core information critical to understanding the topic, while encouraging the reader to look further into the recommended literature.

Through this approach, AOSpine is advancing spine care worldwide.

Luiz Roberto Vialle, MD, PhD

Guest Editors' Preface

The last few decades have seen major advances in our understanding of spinal surgery problems and the options available to diagnose and manage them. Spinal infections can pose challenges in treatment. If there is any delay in diagnosis or if the treatment selected is inappropriate, the result can be serious complications, including intolerable pain, neurological deficit, and progressive deformity. Therefore, it is of utmost importance that the treating physician keep abreast of the latest diagnostic methods and treatment options.

This book is the 10th volume in the successful *AOSpine Masters Series*. It presents an organized and rational approach to the clinical and radiographic evaluation of a patient with spinal infection of whatever etiology. Coverage is exhaustive and includes chapters on epidemiology, pathophysiology, newer diagnostic techniques, conservative treatment, antibiotic therapies, and surgical management. There is also a section on postoperative infections, which present a challenge to every spine surgeon. All of these subjects have been dealt with by renowned spine surgeons with expertise in this field, thereby ensuring that the entire spectrum of knowledge is adequately covered.

This book will be very useful not only for the dedicated spine surgeon but also the orthopaedic generalist who is frequently faced with evaluation and initial treatment of these complicated patients. We are sure that this book will find a place of usefulness on the desk of all spine surgeons from trainees to the most experienced consultant.

S. Rajasekaran, MS ORTHO, FRCS,
FACS, MCh ORTHO, PhD
Rishi M. Kanna, MS, MRCS, FNB SPINE
Giuseppe Barbagallo, MD

Contributors

Abdulaziz Al-Mutair, BHSc, MBChB, FRCS(C)
Consultant Spine Surgeon
AlRazi Orthopedic Hospital, Kuwait
Program Director, Kuwaiti Board of
    Orthopedic Surgery
Kuwait Institute for Medical Specialization
Kuwait

Abdulrazzaq Alobaid, MD, FRCSC
Chairman of the Faculty of Orthopedics
Kuwait Institute for Medical Specialization
Kuwait

Hisam Muhamad Ariffin, MD
Senior Lecture, Consultant Orthopaedic and
    Spine Surgeon
Spine Unit
Department of Orthopaedics
Faculty of Medicine
University of Kebangsaan Malaysia
Faculty of Medicine
Ukm Medical Centre
Cheras, Kuala Lumpur, Malaysia

Hideyuki Arima, MD, PhD
Research Fellow
Norton Leatherman Spine Center
Louisville, Kentucky

Giuseppe Barbagallo, MD
Department of Neurosciences
University of Catania
Catania, Italy

Daniel Beckerman, BA
Research Associate
Department of Orthopaedic Surgery
University of California–San Francisco
San Francisco, California

Sigurd Berven, MD
Professor in Residence
Chief of Spine Service
Department of Orthopaedic Surgery
University of California–San Francisco
San Francisco, California

Joseph S. Butler, PhD, FRCS
Orthopaedic Spine Surgeon
National Spinal Injuries Unit
Mater Misericordiae University
    Hospital
Mater Private Hospital
Tallaght Hospital
Dublin, Ireland

Leah Y. Carreon, MD, MSc
Norton Leatherman Spine Center
Louisville, Kentucky

Robert Dunn, MD
Professor
Department of Orthopaedic Surgery
University of Cape Town and Groote Schuur
    Hospital
Cape Town, South Africa

Mauro Antonio Fernandes, MD
Department of Orthopedics, Spine Unit
Cajuru University Hospital
Catholic University of Parana
Curitiba, Brazil

Steven D. Glassman, MD
Pediatric and Adult Spinal Deformity
    Surgery
Professor of Orthopaedics
Department of Orthopaedic Surgery
University of Louisville School of
    Medicine
Norton Leatherman Spine Center
Louisville, Kentucky

Jeffrey Green, MD
Medical Student
Sydney Kimmel Medical College
Thomas Jefferson University
Philadelphia, Pennsylvania

Alexander V. Gubin, MD
Ministry of Health of the Russian
    Federation Ilizarov Scientific Center
Restorative Traumatology and
    Orthopedics
Kurgan, Russia

Yazeed Gussous, MD
Department of Orthopedics
Ohio State University
Columbus, Ohio

Roger Hartl, MD
Professor
Department of Neurological Surgery
Director of Spinal Surgery
New York Presbyterian Hospital
Weill Cornell Medical College
New York, New York

Christoph-H. Hoffmann, MD
Center for Spinal Surgery and
    Neurotraumatology
BG Unfallklinik
Frankfurt am Main, Germany

Nikhil Jain, MD
Clinical Research Fellow
Division of Spine
Department of Orthopaedics
The Ohio State University
Columbus, Ohio

Frank Kandziora, MD, PhD
Chairman
Center for Spinal Surgery and
    Neurotraumatology
BG-UNfallklink
Frankfurt am Main, Germany

Rishi M. Kanna, MS, MRCS, FNB SPINE
Consultant Spine Surgeon
Ganga Hospital
Coimbatore, India

Yoshiharu Kawaguchi, MD PhD
Clinical Professor
Department of Orthopaedic Surgery
Toyama University Hospital
Toyama, Japan

Diederik Hendrik Ruth Kempen, MD, PhD
Onze Lieve Vrouwe Gasthuis (OLVG)
Amsterdam, The Netherlands

Claudio Lamartina, MD
Istituto Ortopedico Galeazzi
Milan, Italy

Mayan Lendner, BS
Spine Research Fellow
Rothman Institute
Philadelphia, Pennsylvania

Anupama Maheswaran, MBBS
Head
Department of Radiology
Ganga Hospital
Coimbatore, India

Carlotta Martini, MD
Neurosurgeon
Istituto Ortopedico Galeazzi
Milan, Italy

Phelipe de Souza Menegaz, MD
Department of Orthopedics, Spine Unit
Cajuru University Hospital
Catholic University of Parana
Curitiba, Brazil

Hamadi Murphy, MD
Orthopaedic Surgery Resident
Department of Orthopaedic Surgery
School of Medicine
Southern Illinois University
Springfield, Illinois

Alexander Yu. Mushkin, MD
Professor and Head
Pediatric Surgery and Orthopedic Clinic
Coordinator
Nonpulmonary Tuberculosis Direction
St. Petersburg Research Institute of
   Phthisiopulmonology
St. Petersburg, Russia

F. Cumhur Oner, MD, PhD
University Medical Center
Utrecht, The Netherlands

Moritz Perrech, MD
Department of Neurosurgery
University Hospital Cologne
Cologne, Germany

Kris E. Radcliff, MD
Orthopaedic Surgery Attending Physician
   (Spine)
Rothman Institute
Egg Harbor Township, New Jersey

**S. Rajasekaran, MS ORTHO, FRCS, FACS, MCh
   ORTHO, PhD**
Director and Chairman
Department of Orthopaedics & Spine Surgery
Ganga Hospital
Coimbatore, India

Joost P.H.J. Rutges, MD, PhD
Department of Orthopedic Surgery
University Mecical Center
Utrecht, the Netherlands

Klaus John Schnake, MD
Center for Spinal Therapy
Schoen Clinic Nurnberg Fuerth
Fuerth, Germany

Ajoy Prasad Shetty, MS Ortho, DNB Ortho
Consultant Spine Surgeon
Ganga Hospital,
Coimbatore, India

Alexander R. Vaccaro, MD, PhD, MBA
Orthopaedic Surgery Attending Physician
   (Spine)
President
Rothman Institute
Philadelphia, Pennsylvania

Mathew Varghese, MD
Head, Department of Orthopaedics
St. Stephen's Hospital
Tis Hazari, Delhi, India

Alex Vesnaver, MD
Department of Maxillofacial and Oral
   Surgery
University Medical Centre
Ljubljana, Slovenia

Luiz Roberto Vialle, MD, PhD
Professor of Orthopedics, School of
   Medicine
Catholic University of Parana State
Department of Orthopedics, Spine Unit
Cajuru Universitary Hospital
Curitiba, Brazil

ChungChek Wong, MD
Orthopedic Surgeon
Department of Orthopedic Surgery
Sarawak General Hospital
Jalan Tu Ahmad Zaidi Adruce
Kuching, Malaysia

Alberto Zerbi, MD
EFM Professor of Radiology in
   Universities
IRCCS Istituto Ortopedico Galeazzi
Milan, Italy

1

Epidemiology, Microbiology, and Pathology of Spinal Infections

Abdulrazzaq Alobaid and Abdulaziz Al-Mutair

Introduction

Spinal infections are a difficult problem, manifesting either as a dreaded postoperative complication or present as diskitis and osteomyelitis in the absence of previous surgery. Its incidence varies between 1:100,000 and 1:250,000 in developed countries, and its estimated mortality rate ranges between 2% and 4%.[1] The majority of spinal infections are bacterial monomicrobial with an incidence between 30% and 80%.[2–4] Antibiotics are always an important aspect of successful treatment, whether or not surgery is deemed necessary. Establishing the causative organism is of great importance in guiding the selection of the antibiotic and the duration of its administration, because species-specific antibiotics are much preferred over broad-spectrum antibiotics due to optimal efficacy and decreased risk to the patient. Risk factors for spinal infections include poor nutrition, immune suppression, human immunodeficiency virus (HIV) infection, cancer, diabetes, and obesity. Spinal infections can be classified by the anatomic location involved: the vertebral column, intervertebral disk space, the spinal canal, and adjacent soft tissues.

Vertebral osteomyelitis is the most common form of vertebral infection. It can develop from bacteria that spreads to a vertebra, from direct open spinal trauma, and from infections in surrounding areas.

Intervertebral disk space infections involve the space between adjacent vertebrae. Disk space infections can be divided into three subcategories: adult hematogenous (spontaneous), childhood (diskitis), and postoperative.

Spinal canal infections include spinal epidural abscess, which is an infection that develops in the space around the dura (the tissue that surrounds the spinal cord and nerve root). Subdural abscess is far rarer and affects the potential space between the dura and arachnoid (the thin membrane of the spinal cord, between the dura mater and pia mater). Infections within the spinal cord parenchyma (primary tissue) are called intramedullary abscesses.

Adjacent soft tissue infections include cervical and thoracic paraspinal lesions and lumbar psoas muscle abscesses. Soft tissue infections generally affect younger patients and are not seen often in older people. This chapter discusses the epidemiology, microbiology (including brucellosis and tuberculosis), and pathology of spinal infections.

Epidemiology

Spinal infections are among the most troublesome and complex conditions. They may occur in 2 to 7% of patients with musculoskeletal infections.[1,5,6] The incidence peaks in patients younger than 20 years of age and again in patients between 50 and 70 years of age.[2,7] Furthermore, male/female ratios of 2:1 to 5:1 have been reported.[8,9]

Previous spine surgery, a distant infectious focus, diabetes mellitus, advanced age, intravenous drug use, HIV infection, immunosuppression, an oncological history, renal failure, rheumatologic diseases, and liver cirrhosis have been identified as the main predisposing factors.[10,11]

Of late, an increased incidence has been reported, possibly due to the combined effect of an increase in susceptible populations (particularly patients with a history of previous spine surgery) and improved accuracy in diagnosis.[3] Postprocedural diskitis represents up to 30% of all cases of pyogenic spondylodiskitis and has been related to almost all spine surgery techniques.[12,13]

Microbiology

The major agents identified for spinal infections are as follows: bacteria, which cause pyogenic infections; tuberculosis and fungi, which are responsible for granulomatosis infections; less commonly, parasites. With the advances in the diagnosis and treatment of tuberculosis, the incidence of spinal tuberculosis has been reduced, especially in the last 50 years. Bacterial monomicrobial[14,15] spinal infections caused by *Staphylococcus aureus* have an incidence of 30 to 80%.[2-4] Up to 25% of spinal infections are due to gram-negative bacteria such as *Escherichia coli*.[2] *S. aureus* being the most common causative organism, it accounts for about half of all cases.[6] The next most common organism is *Staphylococcus epidermidis*. Gram-negative organisms such as *E. coli* and *Pseudomonas aeruginosa* are less common and seem to be associated with genitourinary infections and procedures as well as with intravenous drug use. Anaerobes are involved rarely. Multiple-organism infections are unusual. Organisms of low virulence, such as skin flora, sometimes are found on culture, and it may be difficult to determine whether they are contaminants or

causative organisms. It should be kept in mind that these organisms can cause vertebral osteomyelitis; therefore, caution should be used when proclaiming them as contaminants.

In HIV-positive patients, *Mycobacterium tuberculosis* accounts for up to 60% of identified pathogens. In cases of penetrating trauma of the spine, anaerobic agents are also a cause of infections.[16] In one third of cases, the infectious agent is never identified.[17,18] Brucellosis and tuberculosis have a high incidence in some endemic areas, such as the Mediterranean countries and in Eastern European countries, and should be given due consideration. Turunc et al,[19] in their prospective study of 75 spondylodiskitis patients, found that tuberculosis was the cause in 13 patients (17.3%), brucellosis was the cause in 32 patients (42.7%), and other bacterial agents were the cause in 30 patients (40%).

Brucellosis is a systemic disease, and many organ systems (e.g., the nervous system, the heart, the skeletal system, and the bone marrow) may become involved following hematogenous dissemination. However, osteoarticular involvement is the most common complication of brucellosis. Osteoarticular involvement has been reported in 10 to 85% of patients in most series.[20] Arthritis and sacroiliitis usually reflect the acute form of brucellosis and frequently respond to the standard therapeutic regimens. In contrast, the spinal column is generally affected in the subacute and chronic forms of brucellosis.[21] Moreover, spinal brucellosis usually affects elderly patients, whereas sacroiliitis and arthritis are usually reported in those in the first three decades of life. The incidence of spinal brucellosis is highly variable (2–54%) depending on the study population.[20] Radiographic abnormalities generally develop 3 to 12 weeks after the onset of clinical symptoms. The spinal column can be affected at any joint, but the lumbar spine is the most commonly involved site, particularly the L4-L5 and L5-S1 junctions.[20] In a review of the literature from Turkey, the authors evaluated 452 spinal brucellosis cases. However, detailed information on the anatomic location of the lesions was available for only 305 cases. Of these lesions, 7% were cervical, 14% were thoracic, 2% were thoracolumbar, 68% were lumbar, 9% were lumbosacral, and 0.3% were sacral. In the majority of patients (98%), a solitary lesion was diagnosed, whereas multiple lesions were diagnosed in only 2%.[6] However, the incidence of multiple site involvement has been reported as 9 to 30%.[22] Abscess formation had rarely been reported in the past, but it has become a common finding (21–42%) following the development of highly sensitive diagnostic techniques such as computed tomography (CT) and magnetic resonance imaging (MRI). The main causes of morbidity in spinal brucellosis are epidural abscess, radiculoneuritis/myelitis, and demyelinating neuropathy.[20]

Pathology

Bacterial infection causing vertebral osteomyelitis can arise from a number of sources. It can occur through direct inoculation, contiguous spread from a nearby infection, or hematogenous seeding. Penetrating injuries and percutaneous or open spinal procedures (e.g., chemonucleolysis, diskography, diskectomy) performed on the intervertebral disk can account for the direct inoculation. Intraabdominal and retroperitoneal abscesses can lead to the local spread of bacteria or fungi. As the number of spinal procedures performed increases, the local spread from direct inoculation of bacteria into the spinal canal becomes more prevalent. But the most common mechanism of spinal infection is still hematogenous seeding of infection. Skin and soft tissue infections, infected vascular access sites, and the urinary tract can be potential sources of pathogenic organisms.

The two major theories for hematogenous dissemination are the venous theory and the arteriolar theory. The venous theory was proposed by Batson,[23] who demonstrated retrograde flow from the pelvic venous plexus to the perivertebral venous plexus via valveless meningorrhachidian veins, using both live animal and human cadaveric models. Wiley and Trueta[24] proposed the arteriolar theory, specifically that bacteria can become lodged in the

end-arteriolar capillary loops. Both mechanisms are likely significant in the establishment of an infectious focus in the spinal column. An extensive prevertebral pharyngeal venous plexus in the cervical spine also may act as a conduit for the spread of bacteria.[25]

There are a variety of ways in which the infection can spread locally. The infection adjacent to the end plate of one vertebral body can rupture through it into the adjoining disk and infect the next vertebral body. The bacterial enzymes can rapidly destroy the relatively avascular disk material. In the cervical spine, the infection can extend into the mediastinum or into the supraclavicular fossa, markedly increasing the extent and severity of the process if it penetrates the prevertebral fascia. Abscess formation from the lumbar spine may track along the psoas muscle and into the buttock (piriformis fossa), the perianal region, the groin, or even the popliteal fossa. The extension of infection from the vertebral body or disk into the spinal canal may result in an epidural abscess or even bacterial meningitis. Destruction of the vertebral body and intervertebral disk can potentially lead to instability and collapse. In addition, with collapse of the vertebral body, infected bone or granulation tissue may be retropulsed into the spinal canal, causing neural compression or vascular occlusion.[26] The lumbar spine is more commonly affected than the thoracic or cervical spine in cases of pyogenic osteomyelitis.[18]

Owing to the anatomic differences in the vascular anatomy of the vertebrae, the pathogenesis of spinal infection differs markedly between children and adults. In children, vascular channels cross the cartilaginous growth plate and end within the nucleus pulposus. These channels provide pathways for direct inoculation of organisms into the vascular nucleus pulposus in children. Due to the absence of these vascular channels in adults, the direct seeding of the disk does not occur, but rather spreading occurs by direct extension with rupture of the infective focus through the end plate into the disk.

A devastating consequence of spinal infection can be neurologic deterioration. A number of factors can cause neural deficit. Direct spread of infected material into the spinal canal can produce an epidural abscess that may compress the neural elements or cause thrombosis or infarction of the regional vascular supply to the spinal cord. Direct hematogenous spread rarely results in epidural abscess without the presence of associated diskitis or osteomyelitis. Pathological fracture can occur, with associated extrusion of either infected material or bony elements into the spinal canal. Kyphosis or spinal instability resulting from destruction of the disk, vertebral bone, and posterior stabilizing structures can cause neural impingement. Diabetes, rheumatoid arthritis, steroid use, advanced age, a more cephalad level of infection (i.e., high thoracic or cervical), and infection with *Staphylococcus* species are some additional risk factors that predispose to neurologic deterioration, as reported by Eismont et al.[27]

The pathophysiology of granulomatous spinal infection differs from that of pyogenic infections. The most common form of granulomatous disease of the spine is caused by *M.tuberculosis* (Pott's disease). Tuberculosis (TB) is endemic in many developing countries, although it has been nearly eradicated in the United States. There has been a recent resurgence of TB with resistant strains in patients with HIV. Although fewer than 10% of patients with TB have skeletal involvement, 50% of the skeletal involvement occurs in the spine. Depending on the series, between 10% and 61% of patients present with or develop a neurologic deficit.[28] With TB, the primary route of infection to the spine is hematogenous from a pulmonary or genitourinary source, although direct spread from adjacent structures can occur. There are three major patterns of spinal vertebral body involvement: peridiskal, central, and anterior.[29] The most common form, peridiskal, occurs adjacent to the vertebral end plate and spreads around a single intervertebral disk. As the granulomatous abscess material tracks beneath the anterior longitudinal ligament, extension to the adjacent vertebra occurs. The second type is central, where infection occurs in the middle of the vertebral body and can be mistaken for a tumor. Destruction of the vertebral body will then lead to spinal deformity. Anterior involvement begins beneath the anterior longitudinal ligament, causing scalloping of the vertebral body. In contrast with peridiskal involvement, which affects a single motion segment, anterior involvement can produce a spinal abscess that extends over multiple levels. Primary involvement of the posterior structures is uncommon. Regionally, the thoracic spine is most often involved, followed by the lumbar spine and cervical spine. Paraspinal extension with abscess formation is common and can occur at any level.

Spinal infections can be classified as acute, subacute, or chronic depending on the duration of symptoms. Symptoms that have persisted for less than 3 weeks are acute, those lasting from 3 weeks to 3 months are subacute, and those lasting more than 3 months are chronic. Chronic infections are caused by indolent organisms, are granulomatous in nature, or are the result of incomplete treatment (e.g., infections with resistant organisms, or the presence of foreign material in the area of infection).

In children, the intraosseous arteries have extensive anastomosis, with some vessels penetrating the intervertebral disk.[30] For this reason, a septic embolus from hematogenous spread does not cause bone infarction, and the infection is located essentially within the disk. The adult intervertebral disk is avascular, and in the third decade of life it undergoes an involution of the intraosseous anastomosis.[31] Therefore, as the adult ages, the release of septic emboli leads to the formation of extensive vascular bone infarcts and the spread of infection to adjacent structures, leading to the classic spondylodiskitis imaging: erosion of vertebral end plates, osteolytic lesions, and compression fractures, which can lead to spine instability, deformity, and the risk of spinal cord compression.[24,31] An infection can lead to uncontrolled spread beyond the bone structures and can access the surrounding tissues, causing paravertebral and psoas abscesses. When spreading into the spinal canal, it can cause epidural abscesses, subdural abscesses, and meningitis. Spreading to the posterior structures is very rare because of its deficit vascular supply and occurs more frequently in fungal and tuberculosis spondylodiskitis.[31]

Pyogenic spondylodiskitis caused by hematogenous spread affects mainly the lumbar spine (58%), followed by the thoracic (30%) and cervical (11%) spines,[14,31] reflecting to some extent the vascular supply of these structures. Tuberculosis lesions preferentially affect the thoracic spine, often involving more than two levels, which differentiates it from pyogenic spondylodiscitis.[14] The direct inoculation pathway is frequently iatrogenic, such as postsurgical lumbar procedures, or after lumbar puncture or epidural procedures.[12] Contiguous spread is rare and may occur in the context of adjacent infection, including esophageal ruptures, retropharyngeal abscesses, or infections of aortic implants.[15]

■ Chapter Summary

Spinal infections remain a rare pathology, although an increased incidence has been reported due to a progressively more susceptible population (particularly in patients with a history of previous spine surgery or who are HIV positive) and improved diagnostic acuity. Due to the insidious onset, a high clinical suspicion remains the centerpiece of a prompt diagnosis, which is pivotal to improve long-term outcomes and prevent permanent neurologic deficits. Microbiological and histological diagnosis plays a critical role in determining therapeutic management. Therefore, following an adequate radiological evaluation of the lesion, CT-guided or open biopsy should be considered the first line of investigation in suspected cases. The treatment of spinal infections is mainly nonsurgical and surgery is indicated for select situations.

Pearls

♦ *Staphylococcus aureus* is the most common causative organism for spinal infection, responsible for about half of all cases.
♦ *Mycobacterium tuberculosis* should always be suspected in HIV-positive patients.

Pitfalls

♦ Organisms of low virulence, such as skin flora, sometimes are found on culture, and it may be difficult to determine whether they are contaminants or causative organisms. It should be kept in mind that these organisms can cause vertebral osteomyelitis; therefore, caution should be used when proclaiming them contaminants.
♦ It is crucial to keep in mind that the pathogenesis of spinal infection differs markedly between children and adults because of anatomic differences in the vascular anatomy of the vertebrae.

References
Five Must-Read References
1. Duarte RM, Vaccaro AR. Spinal infection: state of the art and management algorithm. Eur Spine J 2013; 22:2787–2799
2. Sobottke R, Seifert H, Fätkenheuer G, Schmidt M, Gossmann A, Eysel P. Current diagnosis and treatment of spondylodiscitis. Dtsch Arztebl Int 2008;105: 181–187
3. Jensen AG, Espersen F, Skinhøj P, Rosdahl VT, Frimodt-Møller N. Increasing frequency of vertebral osteomyelitis following Staphylococcus aureus bacteraemia in Denmark 1980–1990. J Infect 1997;34: 113–118
4. Hadjipavlou AG, Mader JT, Necessary JT, Muffoletto AJ. Hematogenous pyogenic spinal infections and their surgical management. Spine 2000;25: 1668–1679
5. Frangen TM, Kälicke T, Gottwald M, et al. [Surgical management of spondylodiscitis. An analysis of 78 cases]. Unfallchirurg 2006;109:743–753
6. Butler JS, Shelly MJ, Timlin M, Powderly WG, O'Byrne JM. Nontuberculous pyogenic spinal infection in adults: a 12-year experience from a tertiary referral center. Spine 2006;31:2695–2700
7. Krogsgaard MR, Wagn P, Bengtsson J. Epidemiology of acute vertebral osteomyelitis in Denmark: 137 cases in Denmark 1978–1982, compared to cases reported to the National Patient Register 1991–1993. Acta Orthop Scand 1998;69:513–517

8. Mylona E, Samarkos M, Kakalou E, Fanourgiakis P, Skoutelis A. Pyogenic vertebral osteomyelitis: a systematic review of clinical characteristics. Semin Arthritis Rheum 2009;39:10–17

9. Grammatico L, Baron S, Rusch E, et al. Epidemiology of vertebral osteomyelitis (VO) in France: analysis of hospital-discharge data 2002–2003. Epidemiol Infect 2008;136:653–660

10. Carragee EJ. Pyogenic vertebral osteomyelitis. J Bone Joint Surg Am 1997;79:874–880

11. Fantoni M, Trecarichi EM, Rossi B, et al. Epidemiological and clinical features of pyogenic spondylodiscitis. Eur Rev Med Pharmacol Sci 2012;16(Suppl 2):2–7

12. Silber JS, Anderson DG, Vaccaro AR, Anderson PA, McCormick P; NASS. Management of postprocedural discitis. Spine J 2002;2:279–287

13. Jiménez-Mejías ME, de Dios Colmenero J, Sánchez-Lora FJ, et al. Postoperative spondylodiskitis: etiology, clinical findings, prognosis, and comparison with nonoperative pyogenic spondylodiskitis. Clin Infect Dis 1999;29:339–345

14. Gouliouris T, Aliyu SH, Brown NM. Spondylodiscitis: update on diagnosis and management. J Antimicrob Chemother 2010;65(Suppl 3):iii11–iii24

15. Babinchak TJ, Riley DK, Rotheram EB Jr. Pyogenic vertebral osteomyelitis of the posterior elements. Clin Infect Dis 1997;25:221–224

16. Lim MR, Lee JY, Vaccaro AR. Surgical infections in the traumatized spine. Clin Orthop Relat Res 2006;444: 114–119

17. Govender S. Spinal infections. J Bone Joint Surg Br 2005;87:1454–1458

18. Sapico FL. Microbiology and antimicrobial therapy of spinal infections. Orthop Clin North Am 1996;27: 9–13

19. Turunc T, Demiroglu YZ, Uncu H, Colakoglu S, Arslan H. A comparative analysis of tuberculous, brucellar and pyogenic spontaneous spondylodiscitis patients. J Infect 2007;55:158–163

20. Alp E, Doganay M. Current therapeutic strategy in spinal brucellosis. Int J Infect Dis 2008;12:573–577

21. Pappas G, Akritidis N, Bosilkovski M, Tsianos E. Brucellosis. N Engl J Med 2005;352:2325–2336

22. Solera J, Lozano E, Martínez-Alfaro E, Espinosa A, Castillejos ML, Abad L. Brucellar spondylitis: review of 35 cases and literature survey. Clin Infect Dis 1999;29:1440–1449

23. Batson OV. The vertebral system of veins as a means for cancer dissemination. Prog Clin Cancer 1967;3: 1–18

24. Wiley AM, Trueta J. The vascular anatomy of the spine and its relationship to pyogenic vertebral osteomyelitis. J Bone Joint Surg Br 1959;41-B:796–809

25. Parke WW, Rothman RH, Brown MD. The pharyngovertebral veins: an anatomical rationale for Grisel's syndrome. J Bone Joint Surg Am 1984;66:568–574

26. Tay BK, Deckey J, Hu SS. Spinal infections. J Am Acad Orthop Surg 2002;10:188–197

27. Eismont FJ, Bohlman HH, Soni PL, Goldberg VM, Freehafer AA. Pyogenic and fungal vertebral osteomyelitis with paralysis. J Bone Joint Surg Am 1983;65: 19–29

28. Boachie-Adjei O, Squillante RG. Tuberculosis of the spine. Orthop Clin North Am 1996;27:95–103

29. Doub HP, Badgley CE. The roentgen signs of tuberculosis of the vertebral body. AJR Am J Roentgenol 1932;27:827–837

30. Ratcliffe JF. An evaluation of the intra-osseous arterial anastomoses in the human vertebral body at different ages. A microarteriographic study. J Anat 1982;134(Pt 2):373–382

31. Ratcliffe JF. Anatomic basis for the pathogenesis and radiologic features of vertebral osteomyelitis and its differentiation from childhood discitis. A microarteriographic investigation. Acta Radiol Diagn (Stockh) 1985;26:137–143

2

Risk Stratification and Prevention of Postoperative Spinal Infections

Hideyuki Arima, Leah Y. Carreon, and Steven D. Glassman

Introduction

The rate of surgical site infection (SSI) in spine surgery has been reported to range from 0.7 to 10.9%.[1,2] Despite an increased focus on risk factors for SSI, infection continues to be major challenge because it is virtually impossible to completely avoid bacterial contamination during surgery. If the host's defense is unable to overcome the bacterial load, SSI may result. Once an infection occurs at the surgical site, treatment requires a substantial use of time and resources, and secondary problems including pseudarthrosis, nerve injury, and poor clinical outcome may result.

In the field of spine surgery, the use of metallic implants has become commonplace. Unfortunately, using instrumentation itself is a risk factor for postoperative SSI as the presence of foreign material suppresses the host's defense locally[3] and helps bacteria in the formation of biofilm.[4] In addition, the use of surgical treatment for elderly people and compromised hosts is increasing. Therefore, risk assessment and precautionary management for postoperative SSI are particularly important in the field of spine surgery. Many risk factors for postoperative SSI have been identified in past studies. Some of these factors are modifiable before surgery and some are not. Recent efforts on the part of spine societies to promote risk stratifi-

cation efforts for SSI after surgery are ongoing. Lee and colleagues[5] developed and validated a predictive model for the risk of SSI after spine surgery based on the patient's comorbidity profile and invasiveness of surgery. We can also predict SSI by using a universal American College of Surgeons National Surgical Quality Improvement Program (ACS-NSQIP) surgical risk calculator.[6] A clearer understanding of preoperative risk for SSI is a necessary condition and first step in optimizing surgical spine care.[7] Also, it is important to mitigate as much as possible the risk factors that can be adjusted. Prevention of postoperative SSI includes both perioperative and postoperative management.

This chapter describes preoperative risk stratification strategies and preventive measures for SSI during surgical preparation, the intraoperative procedure, and postoperative treatment. Postoperative SSI in spine surgery is considered a very serious problem, but unfortunately there are not many high-quality studies in this area. In part, this is due to concerns about the ethical limitations of randomized controlled trials in the field of spine surgery. Therefore, we focused on studies with the highest evidence level based on the appropriate methodology. In studies in which the evidence level is low, we also searched the literature in the field of general orthopedic surgery.

Risk Factors and Risk Stratification for SSI After Spine Surgery

Every operation carries the potential risk of postoperative SSI, because it is very difficult to completely avoid bacterial contamination during surgery. Whether or not the bacterial contamination leads to SSI depends on the quantity and pathogenicity of the bacteria, and on the patients' host defense mechanisms. A relatively large number of studies have identified preoperative factors to help mitigate the risk of SSI. In a systematic review, Pull ter Gunne and colleagues[8] reported 34 variables that are significantly associated with SSI in one or more studies, of which 11 variables were confirmed in two or more studies. These variables can be categorized as patient factors and surgical factors (**Table 2.1**).

Patient Risk Factors

In a study of 24,774 patients enrolled in a prospective registry (Veterans Affairs National Surgical Quality Improvement Program, VA-NSQIP) who underwent spinal decompression and fusion, multivariate logistic regression identified the following risk factors of postoperative SSI: insulin-dependent diabetes; tobacco use; American Society of Anesthesiologists (ASA) class of 3, 4, or 5; a 10% preoperative weight loss in the 6 months before surgery; dependent functional status; and disseminated cancer.[9]

In another systematic review, Schuster and colleagues[10] reported that age > 60 years, presence of diabetes, malnutrition, obesity, ASA score > 3, and higher serum glucose levels were associated with postoperative SSI. In addition, they also described the overall strength of the evidence defining preoperative risk factors for postoperative SSI as "moderate." That is, further research is likely to have an important impact on our confidence in the estimate of effect and may change the estimate. In a more recent systematic review, Pull ter Gunne and colleagues[8] reported that of these variables, only two were found to be significantly related to SSI in more than half of the studies: diabetes mellitus in 11 of 18 studies (61%) and obesity in 8 of 14 studies (57%). They also reported that a history of a spinal infection and ASA risk class were confirmed more often as a significant risk factor for SSI.

A recent general orthopedic study reported on the genetic similarity between nasal *Staphylococcus aureus* isolates and the SSI isolates.[11] Although SSI is generally thought to be caused by bacterial contamination, this study raises the possibility of an endogenous infection pathway. Previous studies reported that preoperative nasal screening test, and sterilization of both nasal cavity and skin in methicillin-resistant *S. aureus* (MRSA) carriers reduced the occurrence of postoperative SSI.[12,13] Verification of this finding in the field of spine surgery is still lacking. Considering the findings from these studies, it is reasonable to acknowledge that diabetes, obesity, ASA grade ≥ 3, history of pre-

Table 2.1 Summary of Various Risk Factors for Surgical Site Infection (SSI) Proposed in the Literature

Patient Factor	Surgical Factor
• Diabetes	• Transfusion
• Obesity	• Posterior approach
• History of previous SSI	
• ASA scores ≥ 3	
• Higher serum glucose levels*	
• Older age	
• Malnutrition*	

*These factors can be modified to mitigate the risk of SSI.

Table 2.2 Summary of Preventive Measures Against SSI Proposed in the Literature

Surgical Preparation	Intraoperative Procedure	Postoperative Treatment
• No shaving	• Application of vancomycin powder to the surgical site	• Early removal of wound drainage
• Use of ultraclean air technology	• Use of dilute povidone-iodine solution as wound irrigation	• Use of silver-impregnated dressings
• Use of double gloving	• Use of antibacterial-coated suture	
• Use of povidone-iodine–containing drapes		
• Assessment protocol		

vious SSI, elevated serum glucose levels, older age, and malnutrition are patient risk factors for SSI (**Table 2.1**).

Surgical Risk Factors

The same VA-NSQIP study reported that fusion/instrumentation, intraoperative transfusion, and an operative duration of longer than 3 hours were significant surgical risk factors for postoperative SSI. Schuster and colleagues[10] reported that blood transfusion and a posterior approach were consistently associated with postoperative SSI. The use of instrumentation and duration of surgery has also been associated with SSI in most studies, but not uniformly. Pull ter Gunne and colleagues[8] noted that while many surgical risk factors have been demonstrated to be significantly associated with the occurrence of an SSI after spine surgery, a causal relationship has less often been confirmed (**Table 2.2**).

Other factors that can be discussed before surgery include the type of surgical approach, the use of microscopes, the staffing requirements in the operating room, geographical variations, and the primary disease being treated.

Risk Stratification and Risk Mitigation

Lee and colleagues[5] published a regression model to predict a patient's risk for postoperative SSI in the field of spine surgery. The postoperative SSI prediction formula is free and available online[14]; the risk factors include heart failure, diabetes, past history of rheumatoid arthritis (RA), surgical invasiveness, older age, diagnosis, weight loss, and obesity. However, these factors are not necessarily consistent with the risk factors identified in previous systematic reviews.[8,10] In addition, the odd ratios for the risk factors were relatively small and may not be clinically relevant.[15] The accuracy of these predictive models may also be influenced by other factors such as the surgeon's skill and the hospital setting. Among the many risk factors for SSI, some variables, such as older age, cannot be modified. However, other variables, such as malnutrition or elevated serum glucose levels, can theoretically be modified to mitigate the risk of SSI.

Preventive Strategies for SSI

Maintaining the surgical site sterility is an important goal in preventing SSI. The strategies to accomplish this goal can be included in the surgical preparation, the intraoperative procedure, and postoperative treatment. We discuss antimicrobial prophylaxis separately.

Surgical Preparation

Shaving

In a randomized trial, Celik and Kara[16] compared the incidence of SSI in a "shaving"cohort (*N* = 371) to a "no shaving" cohort (*N* = 418).

A postoperative infection developed in four patients (1.07%) in the "shaving" group and in one patient (0.23%) in the "no shaving" group ($p < 0.01$). The authors concluded that shaving the patients increases the risk of SSI compared with not shaving them. In addition, current recommendations are to use a surgical clipper, as shaving with a razor with increases the risk of damaging the skin.[17,18]

Surgical Site Scrubbing and Surgical Drape

Although there is no evidence that scrubbing of the surgical site just before surgery is beneficial, it is still recommended in the field of spine surgery. Commonly used disinfectants include chlorhexidine gluconate, povidone iodine, and alcohol. Chlorhexidine gluconate has bactericidal action due to destruction of the cell membrane and has the highest residual effect, but its bactericidal activity against tuberculosis/fungus is somewhat weak, and it takes time to develop its action. Povidone iodine has a bactericidal action due to the oxidizing action of iodine; the residual effect is relatively small, and it takes time to develop its action. Alcohol has a strong bactericidal action due to protein denaturation and is quick acting, but it has no residual effect and is resistant to spores. There is no evidence that scrubbing the surgical site before spine surgery makes a difference in the postoperative SSI incidence.

There is also no evidence that the incidence of postoperative SSI decreases with povidone-iodine–free drape. In general orthopedic surgery, the risk of postoperative SSI may decrease with povidone-iodine–containing drapes.[19] An appropriately powered randomized control study specifically for spine procedures is needed to draw valid conclusions.

Double Gloving

In a prospective study of risk factors for delayed infection, perforation of the glove was identified as a significant risk factor in hip replacement surgery.[20] However, the reduction in SSI by the use of double surgical gloves remains unclear. The rate of inner glove perforation decreases with the use of double surgical glove.[21] Therefore, given the two risks of SSI induction caused by glove perforation and transmission of infection to the surgeon, it is recommended to use double surgical gloves for spine instrumentation surgery.[22]

Surgical Gown

Gowns with nonwoven fabric material may reduce SSI compared with cotton.[23,24] Total body exhaust gowns have been shown to reduce air contamination better than conventional gowns do.[25] But it is still unknown whether total body exhaust gowns will reduce the incidence of postoperative SSI.[26,27] Therefore, at this time, it is not always better to incorporate body exhaust gowns in the spine surgery protocol.

Ultraclean Air Technology and Personnel Traffic in the Operating Room

Because the incidence of SSI correlates with the cleanliness of the operating room, efforts should be made to reduce falling bacteria as much as possible. It is reported that falling bacteria in the operating room is one of the causes of postoperative SSI, and that the number of falling bacteria can be decreased by using the bio-clean room. Only one retrospective cohort study reported a significantly lower postoperative SSI rate in patients undergoing surgery with ultraclean air technology compared with those in conventional operating room conditions in the field of spine surgery (0% versus 12.9%, $p < 0.017$).[28]

The contamination of air in the operating room is influenced by the number of personnel in the room. It is, therefore, important to minimize personnel traffic during surgery. This is also recommended by the Centers for Disease Control and Prevention (CDC) guidelines.[29]

Clinical Assessment Protocol Tool

Christodoulou and colleagues[30] examined the efficiency of using a clinical assessment protocol that addresses patient-related factors, personnel, place, preoperative length of stay, procedure, prosthetics, prophylaxis, packed red blood cells, and pus cultures. They demonstrated that implementation of this clinical assessment protocol significantly reduced the postoperative SSI rate. Vitale and colleagues also proposed regarding SSI prevention strategies as a best practices guideline.[31] Because the evidence level is still low at the present time, further study is necessary.

Intraoperative Procedure

Vancomycin Powder

The direct application of vancomycin powder to the surgical wound has been studied by multiple authors since Sweet and colleagues[32] reported its use in 2011. Although one randomized controlled trial showed local application of vancomycin powder did not significantly reduce the SSI in patients with surgically treated spinal pathologies,[33] two meta-analyses were published in 2014 that concluded that application of vancomycin powder is protective against SSI with a pooled odds ratio (OR) of 0.19 (95% confidence interval [CI], 0.09–0.38)[34] and 0.34 (95% CI, 0.17–0.66).[35] The authors suggested that this benefit may be most appreciated in higher-risk populations or in facilities with a high baseline rate of infection.[35] Godil and colleagues[36] examined the cost-effectiveness of intra-wound vancomycin powder and concluded that the use of vancomycin powder was associated with a significant reduction in both the incidence of postoperative infection and the infection-related medical costs.

Wound Irrigation

In the field of spine surgery, there is no evidence that SSI incidence decreases with wound irrigation with saline solution. But two randomized controlled studies of spine surgery found that wound irrigation with dilute povidone-iodine solution is more effective in preventing postoperative SSI than is irrigation with saline solution.[37,38]

Surgical Suture

It is difficult to conclude what kind of surgical suture the surgeon should use to prevent postoperative SSI. A recent study found that the use of antibacterial-coated suture material decreased postoperative SSI, although surgical numbers were small, and infection rates were low.[39] An appropriately powered randomized controlled study is needed to draw valid conclusions.

Postoperative Treatment

Early Removal of Wound Drains

There is controversy as to whether the use of wound drains reduces the incidence of SSI.[40] The primary indication for using closed suction drains is to decrease the amount of dead space and limit hematoma formation. A retrospective study found that wound drains were left in longer in patients who developed an SSI than in patients who did not (5.1 versus 3.4 days, $p < 0.001$).[41] The authors also reported that the duration of drain placement was an independent risk factor for postoperative SSI in their multivariate analysis (OR, 2.1; 95% CI, 1.6–3.1). If wound drainage is required, closed suction drains are recommended, and it is also recommended to remove the drain as early as possible.[42]

Wound Care

Most spine surgery is clean surgery, and wounds are closed primarily. Therefore, if there is no bleeding or exudate from the surgical site, and the wound barrier is completed, wound care may not be necessary. Currently, wound dressings made of hydrocolloids are considered to be advantageous for wound healing by maintaining a moist environment, but there is no clear evidence that they reduce postoperative SSI. One retrospective cohort study reported a significantly lower postoperative SSI rate in patients treated with silver-impregnated dressings compared with those treated with dry gauze dressings (0% versus 10.9%).[2] Additionally, a prospective analysis of 235 patients undergoing spine surgery reported low postoperative SSI rates in patients treated with 2-octyl-cyanoacrylate for skin closure (0.43%).[43]

Antimicrobial Prophylaxis

Proper Use

Preoperative antimicrobial prophylaxis is suggested to decrease infection rates in patients undergoing spine surgery with or without instrumentation.[44–46] However, despite appropriate prophylaxis, the rate of postoperative SSI in spine surgery is still high (0.7% to 10%).[46–49] Current best practice with antimicrobial prophylaxis protocols has failed to eliminate (i.e., attain an infection rate of 0.0%) postoperative SSI.[44]

Choice of Antibiotics

The published North American Spine Society (NASS) guidelines do not recommend specific antibiotics as antimicrobial prophylaxis for postoperative SSI prevention.[44] The guidelines suggest that antibiotics should be chosen based on the patient's risk factors and allergies, the length and complexity of the procedure, and issues of antibiotic resistance.[44] Generally, in the field of orthopedic surgery, first- and second-generation cephalosporin can be recommended.[50,51] Although the incidence of postoperative SSI by MRSA has been increasing, routine prophylactic administration of MRSA antibiotics cannot be recommended in spine surgery.[44] A meta-analysis in cardiac or orthopedic surgery showed anti-MRSA prophylaxis was significantly protective against SSIs related to MRSA compared with prophylaxis using β-lactam antibiotics (pooled OR, 0.40; 95% CI, 0.20–0.80), and a nonsignificant risk factor for MRSA infections (OR, 1.47; 95% CI, 0.91–2.38).[52] Therefore, prophylactic administration of vancomycin should also be considered at the present time in high-risk patients or in cases of complicated spine surgery.[32,53]

Appropriate Timing and Dose

Because it is important to reach effective blood levels before the procedure, it is necessary to begin intravenous antibiotic prophylaxis 60 minutes prior to the procedure (120 minutes for vancomycin).[50,54–56]

In the NASS guidelines, the particular dose of antimicrobial prophylaxis is not recommended, but it is recommended to administer a standard dose as a single dose in the field of general orthopedic surgery.[50] Considering the low cost and favorable safety profile of cefazolin (a first-generation cephalosporin), increasing the dose to 2 g for patients weighing more than 80 kg and to 3 g for those weighing more than 120 kg can easily be justified.[50]

Re-Dosing and Discontinuation

When cefazolin is used, it is recommended to administer doses every 2 to 4 hours.[50,57] In general, if the surgical time exceeds one to two times the serum half-life of the antibiotic, administering additional doses during the operation should be considered.[42] In the case of vancomycin, additional doses are given in 6 to 12 hours.[50] According to CDC guidelines, it is recommended that the antibiotic be discontinued within 24 hours after the end of surgery.[50]

Chapter Summary

Surgical site infection after spine surgery is difficult to treat. Therefore, it is important to properly recognize the risk factors of SSI. Past studies have identified many patient risk factors for postoperative SSI, including older age, obesity, diabetes, malnutrition, rheumatoid arthritis, nasal MRSA carrier, and high ASA score. Although some of these factors are modifiable, many others are difficult to correct before surgery. In recent years, SSI risk scoring systems have been developed in North America based on the concept of risk stratification. These systems convert the SSI risk for an individual patient with multiple risk factors into an intuitive number (e.g., 5%, 37%). These prediction models also depend on such variables as the surgeon, the surgical facility, and geographical factors, and further research and verification are required. In addition, many elements of peri- and postoperative management aid SSI prevention. Aside from evidence on the use of antibiotic prophylaxis, there are few studies with high levels of evidence on other methods to decrease the incidence of SSI. Further studies will add to the accumulation of evidence in spine surgery.

Pearls

◆ Because it is almost impossible to completely prevent postoperative SSIs, it is important to mitigate SSI by adjusting known risk factors.

◆ By using a prediction model of postoperative SSI risk, the risk for each patient can be determined and a treatment strategy can be selected.
◆ An important strategy is to keep surgical sites sterile to help prevent postoperative SSI.
◆ In spine surgery with or without instrumentation, it is possible to lower the SSI rate by appropriate administration of antimicrobial prophylaxis.

Pitfalls

◆ Performing highly invasive surgery without fully evaluating the risk for postoperative SSI may lead to poor results.
◆ There are still much that we do not know about SSI, so it is necessary to accumulate more evidence in further studies.
◆ Unfortunately, current best practices with antibiotic protocols have failed to eliminate SSIs completely.

References

Five Must-Read References

1. De la Garza-Ramos R, Abt NB, Kerezoudis P, et al. Deep-wound and organ-space infection after surgery for degenerative spine disease: an analysis from 2006 to 2012. Neurol Res 2016;38:117–123
2. Epstein NE. Do silver-impregnated dressings limit infections after lumbar laminectomy with instrumented fusion? Surg Neurol 2007;68:483–485, discussion 485
3. Zimmerli W, Lew PD, Waldvogel FA. Pathogenesis of foreign body infection. Evidence for a local granulocyte defect. J Clin Invest 1984;73:1191–1200
4. von Eiff C, Jansen B, Kohnen W, Becker K. Infections associated with medical devices: pathogenesis, management and prophylaxis. Drugs 2005;65:179–214
5. Lee MJ, Cizik AM, Hamilton D, Chapman JR. Predicting surgical site infection after spine surgery: a validated model using a prospective surgical registry. Spine J 2014;14:2112–2117
6. Bilimoria KY, Liu Y, Paruch JL, et al. Development and evaluation of the universal ACS NSQIP surgical risk calculator: a decision aid and informed consent tool for patients and surgeons. J Am Coll Surg 2013;217:833–42.e1, 3
7. Wang K, Vitale M. Risk stratification: perspectives of the patient, surgeon, and health system. Spine Deform 2016;4:1–2
8. Pull ter Gunne AF, Hosman AJ, Cohen DB, et al. A methodological systematic review on surgical site infections following spinal surgery: part 1: risk factors. Spine 2012;37:2017–2033
9. Veeravagu A, Patil CG, Lad SP, Boakye M. Risk factors for postoperative spinal wound infections after spinal decompression and fusion surgeries. Spine 2009;34:1869–1872
10. Schuster JM, Rechtine G, Norvell DC, Dettori JR. The influence of perioperative risk factors and therapeutic interventions on infection rates after spine surgery: a systematic review. Spine 2010;35(9, Suppl)S125–S137
11. Skråmm I, Fossum Moen AE, Årøen A, Bukholm G. Surgical site infections in orthopaedic surgery demonstrate clones similar to those in orthopaedic Staphylococcus aureus nasal carriers. J Bone Joint Surg Am 2014;96:882–888
12. Price CS, Williams A, Philips G, Dayton M, Smith W, Morgan S. Staphylococcus aureus nasal colonization in preoperative orthopaedic outpatients. Clin Orthop Relat Res 2008;466:2842–2847
13. Gernaat-van der Sluis AJ, Hoogenboom-Verdegaal AM, Edixhoven PJ, Spies-van Rooijen NH. Prophylactic mupirocin could reduce orthopedic wound infections. 1,044 patients treated with mupirocin compared

with 1,260 historical controls. Acta Orthop Scand 1998;69:412–414

14. http://depts.washington.edu/spinersk/generate.php. Accessed Jan. 20, 2017

15. Rochwerg B, Elbarbary M, Jaeschke R, Walter SD, Guyatt GH. Understanding the results: more about odds ratios. In: Guyatt GH, Drummond R, Meade MO, Cook DJ, eds. Users' Guides to the Medical Literature, 3rd ed. New York: McGraw-Hill Education; 2015

16. Celik SE, Kara A. Does shaving the incision site increase the infection rate after spinal surgery? Spine 2007;32:1575–1577

17. Seropian R, Reynolds BM. Wound infections after preoperative depilatory versus razor preparation. Am J Surg 1971;121:251–254

18. Ko W, Lazenby WD, Zelano JA, Isom OW, Krieger KH. Effects of shaving methods and intraoperative irrigation on suppurative mediastinitis after bypass operations. Ann Thorac Surg 1992;53:301–305

19. Ritter MA, Campbell ED. Retrospective evaluation of an iodophor-incorporated antimicrobial plastic adhesive wound drape. Clin Orthop Relat Res 1988; 228:307–308

20. Wymenga AB, van Horn JR, Theeuwes A, Muytjens HL, Slooff TJ. Perioperative factors associated with septic arthritis after arthroplasty. Prospective multicenter study of 362 knee and 2,651 hip operations. Acta Orthop Scand 1992;63:665–671

21. Tanner J, Parkinson H. Double gloving to reduce surgical cross-infection. Cochrane Database Syst Rev 2002:CD003087

22. Savitz SI, Lee LV, Goldstein HB, Savitz MH. Investigations of the bacteriologic factors in cervical disk surgery. Mt Sinai J Med 1994;61:272–275

23. Blomgren G, Hoborn J, Nyström B. Reduction of contamination at total hip replacement by special working clothes. J Bone Joint Surg Br 1990;72:985–987

24. Ahl T, Dalén N, Jörbeck H, Hoborn J. Air contamination during hip and knee arthroplasties. Horizontal laminar flow randomized vs. conventional ventilation. Acta Orthop Scand 1995;66:17–20

25. Sanzén L, Carlsson AS, Walder M. Air contamination during total hip arthroplasty in an ultraclean air enclosure using different types of staff clothing. J Arthroplasty 1990;5:127–130

26. Miner AL, Losina E, Katz JN, Fossel AH, Platt R. Deep infection after total knee replacement: impact of laminar airflow systems and body exhaust suits in the modern operating room. Infect Control Hosp Epidemiol 2007;28:222–226

27. Hooper GJ, Rothwell AG, Frampton C, Wyatt MC. Does the use of laminar flow and space suits reduce early deep infection after total hip and knee replacement?: the ten-year results of the New Zealand Joint Registry. J Bone Joint Surg Br 2011;93:85–90

28. Gruenberg MF, Campaner GL, Sola CA, Ortolan EG. Ultraclean air for prevention of postoperative infection after posterior spinal fusion with instrumentation: a comparison between surgeries performed with and without a vertical exponential filtered airflow system. Spine 2004;29:2330–2334

29. Sehulster L, Chinn RY; CDC; HICPAC. Guidelines for environmental infection control in health-care facilities. Recommendations of CDC and the Healthcare Infection Control Practices Advisory Committee (HICPAC). MMWR Recomm Rep 2003;52(RR-10): 1–42

30. Christodoulou AG, Givissis P, Symeonidis PD, Karataglis D, Pournaras J. Reduction of postoperative spinal infections based on an etiologic protocol. Clin Orthop Relat Res 2006;444:107–113

31. Vitale MG, Riedel MD, Glotzbecker MP, et al. Building consensus: development of a Best Practice Guideline (BPG) for surgical site infection (SSI) prevention in high-risk pediatric spine surgery. J Pediatr Orthop 2013;33:471–478

32. Sweet FA, Roh M, Sliva C. Intrawound application of vancomycin for prophylaxis in instrumented thoracolumbar fusions: efficacy, drug levels, and patient outcomes. Spine 2011;36:2084–2088

33. Tubaki VR, Rajasekaran S, Shetty AP. Effects of using intravenous antibiotic only versus local intrawound vancomycin antibiotic powder application in addition to intravenous antibiotics on postoperative infection in spine surgery in 907 patients. Spine 2013;38: 2149–2155

34. Chiang HY, Herwaldt LA, Blevins AE, Cho E, Schweizer ML. Effectiveness of local vancomycin powder to decrease surgical site infections: a meta-analysis. Spine J 2014;14:397–407

35. Khan NR, Thompson CJ, DeCuypere M, et al. A meta-analysis of spinal surgical site infection and vancomycin powder. J Neurosurg Spine 2014;21:974–983

36. Godil SS, Parker SL, O'Neill KR, Devin CJ, McGirt MJ. Comparative effectiveness and cost-benefit analysis of local application of vancomycin powder in posterior spinal fusion for spine trauma: clinical article. J Neurosurg Spine 2013;19:331–335

37. Chang FY, Chang MC, Wang ST, Yu WK, Liu CL, Chen TH. Can povidone-iodine solution be used safely in a spinal surgery? Eur Spine J 2006;15:1005–1014

38. Cheng MT, Chang MC, Wang ST, Yu WK, Liu CL, Chen TH. Efficacy of dilute betadine solution irrigation in the prevention of postoperative infection of spinal surgery. Spine 2005;30:1689–1693

39. Ueno M, Saito W, Yamagata M, et al. Triclosan-coated sutures reduce wound infections after spinal surgery: a retrospective, nonrandomized, clinical study. Spine J 2015;15:933–938

40. Payne DH, Fischgrund JS, Herkowitz HN, Barry RL, Kurz LT, Montgomery DM. Efficacy of closed wound

suction drainage after single-level lumbar laminectomy. J Spinal Disord 1996;9:401–403

41. Rao SB, Vasquez G, Harrop J, et al. Risk factors for surgical site infections following spinal fusion procedures: a case-control study. Clin Infect Dis 2011;53: 686–692

42. Mangram AJ, Horan TC, Pearson ML, Silver LC, Jarvis WR; Hospital Infection Control Practices Advisory Committee. Guideline for prevention of surgical site infection, 1999. Infect Control Hosp Epidemiol 1999; 20:250–278, quiz 279–280

43. Wachter D, Brückel A, Stein M, Oertel MF, Christophis P, Böker DK. 2-Octyl-cyanoacrylate for wound closure in cervical and lumbar spinal surgery. Neurosurg Rev 2010;33:483–489

44. Shaffer WO, Baisden JL, Fernand R, Matz PG; North American Spine Society. An evidence-based clinical guideline for antibiotic prophylaxis in spine surgery. Spine J 2013;13:1387–1392

45. Barker FG II. Efficacy of prophylactic antibiotic therapy in spinal surgery: a meta-analysis. Neurosurgery 2002;51:391–400, discussion 400–401

46. Hellbusch LC, Helzer-Julin M, Doran SE, et al. Single-dose vs multiple-dose antibiotic prophylaxis in instrumented lumbar fusion—a prospective study. Surg Neurol 2008;70:622–627, discussion 627

47. Rubinstein E, Findler G, Amit P, Shaked I. Perioperative prophylactic cephazolin in spinal surgery. A double-blind placebo-controlled trial. J Bone Joint Surg Br 1994;76:99–102

48. Rechtine GR, Bono PL, Cahill D, Bolesta MJ, Chrin AM. Postoperative wound infection after instrumentation of thoracic and lumbar fractures. J Orthop Trauma 2001;15:566–569

49. Kanayama M, Hashimoto T, Shigenobu K, Oha F, Togawa D. Effective prevention of surgical site infection using a Centers for Disease Control and Prevention guideline-based antimicrobial prophylaxis in lumbar spine surgery. J Neurosurg Spine 2007;6: 327–329

50. Bratzler DW, Houck PM; Surgical Infection Prevention Guidelines Writers Workgroup; American Academy of Orthopaedic Surgeons; American Association of Critical Care Nurses; American Association of Nurse Anesthetists; American College of Surgeons; American College of Osteopathic Surgeons; American Geriatrics Society; American Society of Anesthesiologists; American Society of Colon and Rectal Surgeons; American Society of Health-System Pharmacists; American Society of PeriAnesthesia Nurses; Ascension Health; Association of periOperative Registered Nurses; Association for Professionals in Infection Control and Epidemiology; Infectious Diseases Society of America; Medical Letter; Premier; Society for Healthcare Epidemiology of America; Society of Thoracic Surgeons; Surgical Infection Society. Antimicrobial prophylaxis for surgery: an advisory statement from the National Surgical Infection Prevention Project. Clin Infect Dis 2004;38:1706–1715

51. Nishant, Kailash KK, Vijayraghavan PV. Prospective randomized study for antibiotic prophylaxis in spine surgery: choice of drug, dosage, and timing. Asian Spine J 2013;7:196–203

52. Schweizer M, Perencevich E, McDanel J, et al. Effectiveness of a bundled intervention of decolonization and prophylaxis to decrease gram positive surgical site infections after cardiac or orthopedic surgery: systematic review and meta-analysis. BMJ 2013;346: f2743

53. Klekamp J, Spengler DM, McNamara MJ, Haas DW. Risk factors associated with methicillin-resistant staphylococcal wound infection after spinal surgery. J Spinal Disord 1999;12:187–191

54. Milstone AM, Maragakis LL, Townsend T, et al. Timing of preoperative antibiotic prophylaxis: a modifiable risk factor for deep surgical site infections after pediatric spinal fusion. Pediatr Infect Dis J 2008;27:704–708

55. Olsen MA, Nepple JJ, Riew KD, et al. Risk factors for surgical site infection following orthopaedic spinal operations. J Bone Joint Surg Am 2008;90:62–69

56. Bratzler DW, Dellinger EP, Olsen KM, et al; American Society of Health-System Pharmacists; Infectious Disease Society of America; Surgical Infection Society; Society for Healthcare Epidemiology of America. Clinical practice guidelines for antimicrobial prophylaxis in surgery. Am J Health Syst Pharm 2013;70: 195–283

57. Ohge H, Takesue Y, Yokoyama T, et al. An additional dose of cefazolin for intraoperative prophylaxis. Surg Today 1999;29:1233–1236

3

Imaging in Spinal Infections

Anupama Maheswaran and Alberto Zerbi

Introduction

Spinal infections are serious disorders, and it is imperative that the diagnosis be achieved as early as possible. Delay in appropriate treatment can result in irreversible sequelae such as instability, incapacitating deformity, and neurologic deficit.[1] Imaging plays a vital role, as it provides valuable information regarding the presence and location of infection, the severity of disease, associated morphological changes, and clues toward the causative organism.[2]

Although plain radiography remains the basic modality of investigation, advanced imaging techniques aid in early and accurate detection of radiographically occult, multifocal, and skip lesions.[3,4] They also enable tissue sampling at the most representative site within the lesion. In recent times, imaging is also increasingly used to assess the response and healing status of spinal infections after treatment.[5]

The imaging techniques include plain radiography, ultrasonography (USG), computed tomography (CT), magnetic resonance imaging (MRI), and nuclear scintigraphy scans. Each technique has advantages and limitations (**Table 3.1**). It is imperative that the techniques be skillfully used to the benefit of the patient. The treating physician and radiologist must also be aware of conditions such as degenerative spondylitis, inflammatory spondylitis, and neuropathic spondylo-arthropathy that can often mimic infection; in those situations, imaging should be interpreted with caution.

Pathophysiology

The commonest mode of infection in the spine is by hematogenous seeding of microorganisms, either through arterial arcades or venous plexus.[6] Retrograde flow of blood from the pelvic venous plexus to the perivertebral venous plexus has been demonstrated and is believed to be a major conduit for spread of infections.[7] Other modes of infection include iatrogenic direct inoculation and spread of infection from adjacent sites.[8] The frequent sites of pyogenic spondylodiskitis are the lower thoracic and lumbar spine followed by the upper thoracic region.[9] For tuberculosis (TB), the thoracic spine (37.5%) is the commonest location, followed by the thoracolumbar region (27.5%).[10]

The intervertebral disks in children remain vascular up to 7 years of age, allowing primary inoculation of infection in the disk. After 7 to 8 years of age, hematogenous infections primarily infect the subchondral bone, with secondary involvement of the disks. Paradiskal infection on either side of the disk is the most common pattern of infection, as embryologically the disk and the adjacent bodies are supplied by the branches of the same vessel.[11] Marrow signal

Table 3.1 Various Imaging Modalities in the Evaluation of Spinal Infections

Imaging	Advantages	Disadvantages
X-ray	• Portable • Cheap	• Detects only advanced disease
CT	• Less time-consuming • Best spatial resolution • Good cortical bone visualization • Posterior elements better delineated • Field of view can be increased to include adjacent areas • Useful in junctional regions • Multiplanar reconstruction and 3D reformation guide surgical planning	• Exposure to ionizing radiation, and hence usage is restricted in children • Pregnancy is a relative contraindication
MRI	• Gold standard • Best soft tissue resolution • Early detection • Better visualization of cord, bone marrow, disk, ligaments, facet joints, thecal sac, epidural and paravertebral soft tissues • No radiation hazard • Whole spine MRI helps in identifying asymptomatic skipped lesions • Interval MRI is useful to assess disease healing	• Limited availability • Expensive • Acoustic noise (65 to 95 dB) • Time-consuming • Claustrophobia • Contraindicated for patients with foreign bodies near the orbit, such as pacemakers, cochlear implants, external fixators, and aneurysmal clips • Metal artifacts, due to implants, are challenging in postoperative cases
Scintigraphy	• Earliest modality to detect infection • High sensitivity (as high as 95%)	• False-negative results in lesions that are purely lytic, involving isolated neural arch, or avascular, involving cervical spine or disseminated lesions • Low specificity and lack of spatial resolution
PET CT	• Useful in follow-up study to assess the treatment response and healing • Carbon-11 choline PET used to differentiate infection and malignancy	• Expensive • Limited availability • Significant false-positive results

Abbreviations: CT, computed tomography; MRI, magnetic resonance imaging; PET, positron emission tomography; 3D, three-dimensional.

alteration due to increased water content by exudates and edema is the earliest radiological finding detected by MRI, much before the appearance of radiographic changes.[12] In TB, four types have been described based on the location of the lesion: paradiskal, central, anterior, and appendicular.[13]

Pyogenic organisms release proteolytic enzymes such as hyaluronic acid, which destroy the disk substance early. With advancing subchondral infection, the intervening disk loses its nutrition, and this leads to secondary destruction with loss of disk height.[14] In contrast, disk involvement is late in mycobacterial infections due to the lack of proteolytic enzymes. The hypersensitive response of the host leading to marked exudation with an abscess containing inflammatory cells, caseous material, bone fragments, and occasionally tubercle bacilli can cause a large abscess in TB.[15]

The constant increase in life expectancy and the ever-increasing incidence of medical comorbidities such as diabetes mellitus, hypertension, and HIV infections, along with the high prevalence of immune-deficient survivors, have resulted in an overall global increase in spinal infections.[16] In addition, with increasing reliance on surgical management of spinal disorders, iatrogenic and postoperative spinal infections have also become a cause of concern.[17]

Plain Radiography

Plain radiography is the primary investigation of choice, but it has the limitation of delayed diagnosis of even up to 6 months, as at least 30% of bone destruction is required for identification.[5] Furthermore, lesions of the sacrum, neural arch/facet joints, and craniovertebral and cervicothoracic junctions could go undetected on radiographs.

Radiographic findings suggestive of infection include reduction in disk space, demineralization with blurring, resorption/erosion of end plates, and destruction and collapse of the vertebral body, resulting in deformity[18] (**Figs. 3.1** and **3.2**). Indirect evidence of infections is the presence of prevertebral soft tissue shadows of abscesses in the cervical spine and thickened paravertebral shadows at the thoracolumbar region. Erosions in the anterior and lateral aspect of the vertebral body, called the Gouge defect, occur due to an anterior subperiosteal lesion under the anterior longitudinal ligament.[19] The aneurysmal phenomenon or syndrome represents anterior marginal scalloping, which is due to the mass effect.[20] Although a large anterior collection of abscesses is the usual cause, it can also be due to lymphomas or aortic aneurysms. In advanced thoracic spine lesions with collapse, a bird's-nest appearance due to radiodense globular and fusiform shadows can be seen.[21] There are no concrete radiographic features to differentiate pyogenic and TB spondylitis. However, the involvement of more than two vertebral bodies and the presence of perivertebral abscesses are more common in TB.

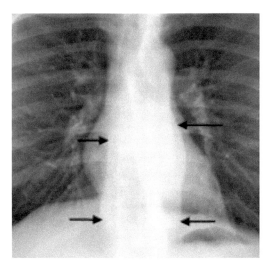

Fig. 3.1 A frontal projection of a chest radiograph demonstrating an early radiographic feature of infective spondylitis at the thoracolumbar junction: a displaced posteromedial pleural line *(black arrows)* representing a paravertebral "petering abscess," which shows a converging yet indistinct lower border.

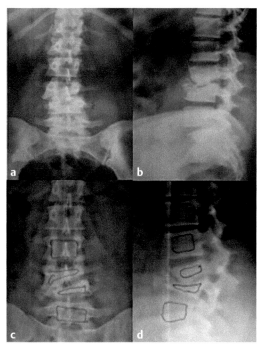

Fig. 3.2 Lumbar spine radiographs in infective spondylodiskitis: **(a)** anteroposterior (AP) view and **(b)** lateral view demonstrate destruction of the disk space and end plates. **(c,d)** Corresponding follow-up radiographs demonstrate progressive bony destruction and collapsed vertebral bodies.

Computed Tomography Scan

The CT scan has the advantage of early detection of infection when compared with plain radiography, but it cannot detect the subchondral marrow changes that are seen on MRI, which are the earliest signs of infection. CT clearly demonstrates the bony morphology, the extent of osseous destruction, bone fragmentation, calcification in soft tissues, and the extent of deformity (**Fig. 3.3**). Since CT provides irrefutable detail in evaluating the anatomy of the facets, pedicles and lamina, it helps the surgeon to decide on the need for instrumentation based on the stability of the spine. Bone fragments can be detected in the epidural soft tissue collections too (**Fig. 3.3f**). Air pockets due to gas collection can be seen at the site of infection (**Fig. 3.3e**) and is referred to as emphysematous osteomyelitis of the spine.

A plain CT does not demonstrate epidural involvement or spinal cord compression. CT myelogram is useful in detecting spinal canal compromise. Contrast-enhanced CT defines the extent of tubercular abscess, but the extent of epidural involvement cannot be determined. The CT features that suggest pyogenic spondylodiskitis include moderate circumferential paravertebral soft tissue involvement, sparing of posterior appendages, gas within the bone, disk space narrowing, and diffuse bone destruction.[22] Four patterns of bone destruction have been described in TB: osteolytic, fragmentary, subperiosteal, and localized sclerotic lesions (**Fig. 3.3**). The fragmentary type is most common (47%), followed by the lytic type (24.1%).[23]

Magnetic Resonance Imaging

Magnetic resonance imaging is the most sensitive of all diagnostic investigations and is also the imaging modality of choice in spinal infections.[24] It is noninvasive, and it is safer than both CT and plain radiography in that MRI does not employ harmful ionizing radiations.

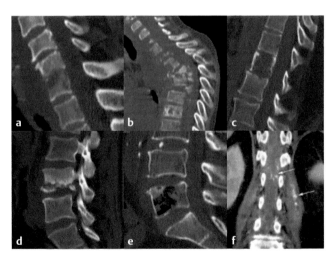

Fig. 3.3 Multiplanar sagittal reconstructed computed tomography (CT) images demonstrate several different patterns in infective spondylodiskitis: **(a)** destruction of the disk space and end plates, **(b)** multilevel extensive bony destruction and collapsed vertebral bodies with several bone fragments seen extending into the epidural and paravertebral soft tissue abscess with advanced kyphotic deformity, **(c)** predominantly lytic pattern, **(d)** lytic pattern with adjacent sclerosis, **(e)** emphysematous osteomyelitis of L5 vertebral body with intraosseous air pockets, and **(f)** calcification in the paravertebral and intraspinal soft tissue components.

Although whole spine CT is harmful, whole spine MRI is safe and aids in detecting satellite and skip lesions efficiently. In addition, it enables detailed evaluation of the vertebral marrow, the disk space, the neural arch, the facet joint, paravertebral and epidural soft tissue, and the intraspinal structures including the dura, nerve roots, and the cord. MRI offers the benefit of analyzing the sacroiliac joints too, which if involved do not produce obvious radiographic changes.

The MRI sequences taken during evaluation of spinal infections include T1-weighted imaging (T1WI), T2-weighted imaging (T2WI), short tau inversion recovery (STIR) sequences, and contrast-enhanced T1WI. Marrow edema is the earliest sign that can be detected, and it appears hypointense on T1WI, isointense on T2WI, and hyperintense on STIR sequences (**Fig. 3.4**).[25] The STIR sequence (a type of fat-suppression sequence) is the most sensitive in detecting marrow edema (**Fig. 3.5**).[3] In spinal infections, the usual pattern observed is the involvement of two adjoining vertebrae and the intervening disk. However, the collapse of a vertebral body with intraosseous abscess or bony destruction is not uncommon. Altered morphology of the disk can also be seen with loss of differentiation of the annulus fibrosus and nucleus pulposus, effacement of the intradiskal nuclear cleft, the appearance of intradiskal collection, and progressive reduction in its height (**Figs. 3.6** and **3.7**).

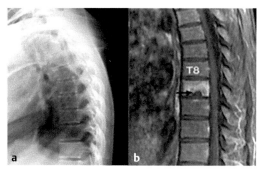

Fig. 3.4 (a) Lateral radiograph of the thoracic spine appears normal. **(b)** Contrast-enhanced magnetic resonance imaging (MRI) with a sagittal T1-weighted image (T1WI) shows abnormal enhancement *(arrow)* of the T8 vertebral body with destruction of the inferior end plate, consistent with early spondylitis.

Tuberculous versus Pyogenic Infection

Differentiation of tubercular and pyogenic lesions can be challenging. The thoracolumbar spine is the most common region affected in TB as compared with lumbar spine involvement in pyogenic infections.[26] In TB, the involvement of the cervical spine and the isolated neural arch or facet joint is extremely rare. Involvement of the unilateral lamina and spinous process of the cervical and upper thoracic regions, although rare, is relatively frequent in

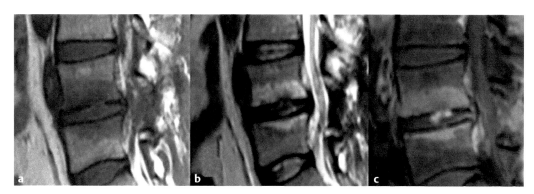

Fig. 3.5 Sagittal MRI sections with characteristic imaging findings of early diskitis shows altered signal intensities in the subchondral bone of the adjacent vertebral bodies and intervening disk: **(a)** hypointense on T1 weighted image, **(b)** isointense on T2-weighted image, and **(c)** enhancement in T1-weighted image fat-suppressed postcontrast sequence.

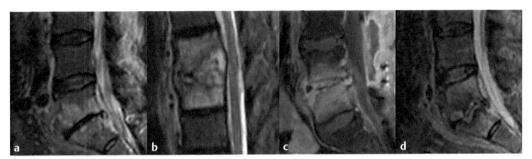

Fig. 3.6 Sagittal MRI scans of four patients with characteristic findings of infective spondylodiskitis: **(a)** loss of nuclear cleft, **(b)** extension of marrow edema greater than one half of the vertebral body with irregular margins, **(c)** end plate erosions, and **(d)** intradiskal high signal with loss of disk height.

TB, whereas facet joint and adjacent articular facets are more often involved in pyogenic spondylitis.[27] The diagnostic clues in differentiating TB from pyogenic infection are listed in **Table 3.2**.[28]

The MRI features of TB may be typical or atypical, and with the increasing incidence of multidrug-resistant strains, atypical clinical and radiological presentations are on the rise. Subligamentous spread of inflammatory tissue and initial preservation of the disk spaces are characteristic features of TB. Typical TB spondylitis is seen affecting a single region in ~ 65% of patients. Multiple contiguous-level infections are seen in 20% and multiple noncontiguous skip levels of involvement in ~ 10% (**Table 3.2**). Atypical radiological presentations of spinal TB include osseous destruction of the vertebral body with sparing of the disks (**Fig. 3.8**); vertebra plana (advanced collapse of the vertebral body), which is more common in children; ivory vertebra; isolated involvement of the neural arch/facet joint; a solid soft tissue component; and noncontiguous bony lesions (**Fig. 3.8c**).

Soft Tissue Involvement and Abscess Formation

Soft tissue involvement can be either be in the form of phlegmon or an abscess formation in the epidural, paravertebral, or paraspinal regions. The common locations of abscesses are the subligamentous, psoas, and paraspinal muscles in the thoracolumbar spine; pleural empyema in the thoracic region; and retropharyngeal abscess in the cervical spine. Smaller abscesses with thick irregular walls are frequently seen in pyogenic infections.[29] Abscesses are better delineated on T2WI scans. They appear as loculated and well-encapsulated collections with

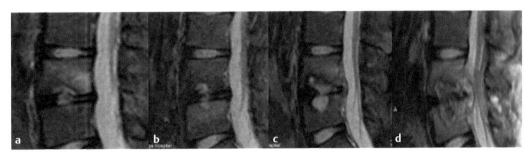

Fig. 3.7 Serial follow-up sagittal MRI scans of a 45-year-old man diagnosed with infective spondylodiskitis and started on antibiotic therapy, showing progression of spondylodiskitis from **(a)** subchondral bone marrow edema to **(b)** end plate erosion, **(c)** disk involvement, and **(d)** appearance of an epidural abscess.

Table 3.2 Differentiation of Tuberculosis and Pyogenic Spondylodiskitis

Characteristic	Tuberculosis	Pyogenic
Bone destruction	50–75%	< 50%
Thoracic spine involvement	40% with or without kyphosis	10%, lumbar more common
Vertebral bodies involvement	Solitary, collapse, skip, contiguous of more than three bodies	Ill-defined end plates with erosions
Neural arch involvement	Rare, pedicle and lamina	Rare, facet joints
Disk	Relative sparing or late involvement	Early disk involvement, rapid loss of disk height
Enhancement of vertebral body	Inhomogeneous	Homogeneous
Enhancement of soft tissues	Well-defined smooth peripheral	Ill-defined, thick wall in 9%
Well-defined paravertebral collection	95%	25%
Thin, smooth wall of abscess	95%	15%
Paravertebral or intraosseous abscess	95%, large	50%, small
Subligamentous spread along three or more vertebral bodies	85%	40%
Computed tomography	More common calcification, in wall of soft tissue abscess Bone fragment within lytic lesions and sclerotic margins Larger end-plate erosions	Rare

thin, smooth walls and are usually isointense to cerebrospinal fluid (CSF) in all sequences with homogeneously hyperintense signals on T2WI and hypointense signals on T1WI (**Fig. 3.9**).

Contrast Magnetic Resonance Imaging

Intravenous administration of gadolinium-based contrast medium (0.1 mmol/kg body weight) is useful in select cases. Enhancement of involved marrow, disk, and soft tissues can be seen in postcontrast T1WI fat-suppressed images (**Fig. 3.9**). Homogeneous enhancement in paravertebral or epidural soft tissue indicates granulation tissue and phlegmon forma-

tion.[15] The "rind sign" has been described for peripheral rim enhancement of the abscess with a nonenhancing central portion that has undergone caseous necrosis (**Fig. 3.10**).[30]

Intraspinal Infections

Intraspinal infections can be epidural, subdural, or intradural. Although epidural lesions are common among the three types, an isolated epidural abscess is extremely rare and is usually secondary to remote infection in the disk or the facet joint (**Fig. 3.10**). Epidural abscess, especially pyogenic, can cause significant canal stenosis and compression of the cord or nerve roots, and is considered a surgical emergency.[31] Neurologic deficit in an intraspinal infection is

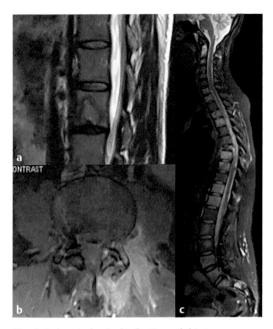

Fig. 3.8 Atypical spinal infections: **(a)** intraosseous abscess in a vertebral body in a sagittal T2WI, **(b)** facetitis with left paraspinal soft tissue enhancement in postcontrast T1WI fat-suppressed axial image, **(c)** skip lesions in T2 suppressed whole sagittal MRI.

either due to direct compression of the cord by an abscess or inflammatory tissue. It may also occur as a response to an adjacent infection causing secondary myelitis or infarction, which can be detected by MRI.[32] Intradural infection can involve the meninges or cord and rarely

may present as intramedullary tuberculoma or cord abscess.

Although thecal sac compression by epidural lesions can be well visualized on magnetic resonance myelography, spinal cord involvement is best evaluated with MRI on T2WI and postcontrast T1WI. Tuberculoma can be seen within the cord as a ring or patchy enhancing lesion with surrounding edema, which can mimic tumor.[33] Meningeal involvement can also be diagnosed by MRI. Arachnoiditis is one of the common complications of intraspinal infection and can be detected easily by MRI, which reveals clumping of nerve roots in the early stages, and then may lead to leptomeningeal adhesions causing angular defects in the dural sac, and finally to peripheral adherence of the nerve roots to the thecal sac, resulting in the characteristic "empty sac" sign.[34] A bulky cord with ill-defined mild hyperintense signal on T2WI suggests cord edema, which has a favorable prognosis. In contrast, a reduced caliber with bright signal of the cord implies myelomalacia and it indicates a poor recovery.

Nuclear Imaging

Scintigraphic scans are usually done with technetium-99m diphosphonate as a tracer administered intravenously, followed by three-phase bone scans. Nuclear scans are believed to be able to indicate a possible infection earlier than

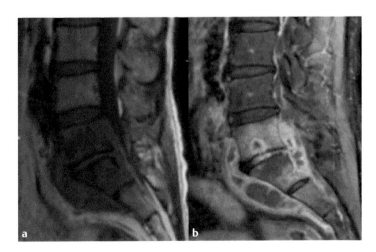

Fig. 3.9 Sagittal MRI sections: **(a)** T1WI and **(b)** postcontrast T1 fat-suppressed section showing marrow edema of adjacent bodies, enhancing disk, and rim enhancement of epidural and prevertebral abscesses suggestive of infective spondylodiskitis.

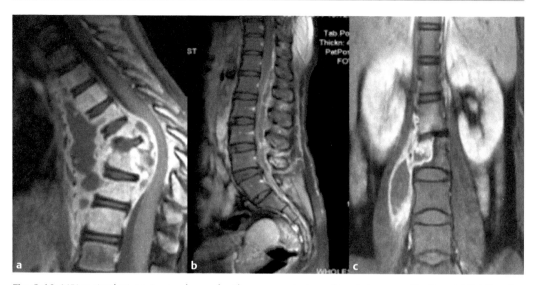

Fig. 3.10 MRI sagittal T1 contrast enhanced with fat suppression images of three patients: **(a)** multi-level contiguous involvement of the midthoracic vertebrae with associated collapse, kyphosis, and subligamentous and epidural abscesses; **(b)** isolated posterior epidural abscess collection; **(c)** Pott's spine with isolated vertebral body involvement with mild destruction and right lateral wedging. Peripheral smooth thin rim enhancement of abscesses is also seen.

any other imaging technique, as early as within 48 hours of onset of symptoms.[35] However, the lack of resolution and its poor specificity has restricted its use to only ambiguous cases. Gallium-67 citrate and indium-111–labeled autologous white blood cell scintigraphy have a better specificity and are useful in the setting of pyrexia of unknown origin.[36]

Fluorodeoxyglucose (FDG) positron emission tomography (PET) is more useful in assessing metabolic activity of the lesion by analyzing the standardized uptake values (SUVs); the activity is considered high if the SUV is greater than 2.5.[37] However, an elevated SUV can also be noted in malignancy and granulomatous diseases such as TB, sarcoidosis, histoplasmosis, and aspergillosis. Delayed scans may be useful in differentiating TB and malignancy. In both cases, the SUV peaks at around 60 minutes; later activity declines or becomes stabilized in TB, whereas it tends to increase in malignancy.[38] Quantitative PET-CT scans are thought to be useful when the MRI findings are equivocal, and are early surrogate markers of treatment response in TB. Carbon-11 choline PET has also been used to differentiate infection and malignancy.[39]

Image-Guided Diagnostic and Therapeutic Procedures

Imaging guidance by fluoroscopy, CT, or ultrasound can be used appropriately for procedures such as biopsy, aspiration, local instillation of antibiotics, and pigtail insertion for percutaneous drainage of abscesses. Apart from increasing the diagnostic accuracy and efficacy, it is also cost-effective, faster, safe, and minimally invasive.[40] In addition, it can be done as an outpatient procedure, with avoidance of injury to neural and vascular structures.[41] Although this is a minimally invasive procedure with acceptable yield rates, some centers use open biopsy instead, as it allows the surgeon to obtain adequate sampling tissue and to do a debridement/decompression and stabilization procedure at the same time.

The role of ultrasonography is limited in making the initial diagnosis, but it can be used as a screening procedure for large iliopsoas abscess, and it aids in both biopsy sampling and percutaneous aspiration/drainage of abscess.[42] Bleeding parameters have to be checked before biopsy and percutaneous drainage of abscess. Aspirating an abscess helps to reduce inflammation and promote healing. It also relieves discomfort for the patient, especially when an iliopsoas abscess causing a pseudo–hip flexion deformity is being drained. Cutting needles (10 to 14 G) are generally used for biopsy and smaller needles (18 to 21 G) for aspiration. The coaxial technique enables local anesthetic administration and passage of biopsy needles multiple times with a single superficial skin puncture, thus increasing the diagnostic yield, and it has fewer complications. Pigtail catheters (6 to 8 F) are used for drainage of large abscess and are connected to an airtight bag. The aspirated samples are taken in sterile containers and sent to the laboratory for microbiological and histopathological analysis. The puncture site should be monitored for any worrisome bleeding, and the patients are usually observed for 2 to 4 hours following the procedure depending on the type of anesthesia.

Infective Spondylodiskitis in Postoperative Cases

The incidence of postoperative spinal infection varies from 1 to 3%. Unlike the hematogenous spread of tubercular and pyogenic infections, this is most often due to direct inoculation. It is difficult to assess postoperative spinal infections due to magnetic susceptibility artifacts on MRI and streak artifacts on CT because of implants with obscuration of image details.[43] The possibility of postoperative infection is considered if there are new erosions of the end plate, osteolysis, marrow edema, and intradiskal or epidural abscess. A migrated hardware component (**Fig. 3.11**), peri-implant collection, and loosening of screws are indirect evidence of infection (**Fig. 3.12**).[44] Intraspinal and paraspinal abscess are identified with rim enhancement of the collections (**Fig. 3.13**). Contrast MRI is the investigation of choice in diagnosing postoperative spinal infection, and it enables differentiating edema and infection.[45]

Assessment of Response to Treatment

With increasing instances of antibiotic-resistant microorganisms and multidrug tuberculosis resistance, it is absolutely necessary for the physician to use the appropriate antibiotics at adequate doses for a safe period of time. Chronic usage of antibiotics is not recommended unless warranted in specific cases. Antitubercular drugs have multiple side effects and must be used judiciously. Henceforth, treatment in spinal infections should be tailored individually and requires modifications based on the treatment response. The current recommendation of antibiotic duration is 6 weeks for pyogenic infection and 6 to 9 months for tuberculosis.

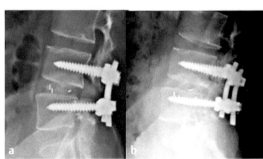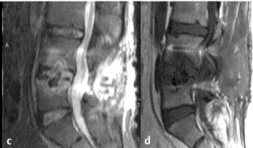

Fig. 3.11 Postoperative infections: **(a)** lateral radiograph shows postoperative status with L4–5 posterior instrumented stabilization and an interbody peek cage in situ. **(b)** Two-month follow-up lateral radiograph shows subsidence of the cage.

Further evaluation by MRI with **(c)** T1WI and **(d)** T2WI sagittal sections shows the underlying cause as diskitis with altered signal in the disk, inferior settling of the interbody cage, subchondral marrow edema, and end-plate erosions.

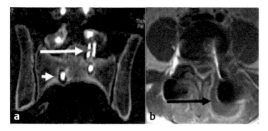

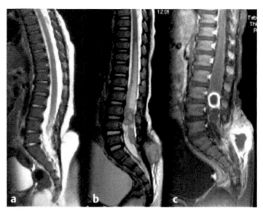

Fig. 3.12 Postoperative infections: **(a)** reformatted coronal CT image shows a migrated cage displaced to the left neural foramen *(long white arrow)* and loosening of pedicle screw with surrounding lucency *(short white arrow)*. **(b)** In another postoperative case, an axial T1WI scan shows the implant rendering magnetic susceptibility artifacts, and a thin-walled collection *(black arrow)* around the left pedicle screw and epidural region posteriorly.

Fig. 3.13 Postoperative infection in a 2-year-old child who underwent surgery for a tethered cord. **(a)** Preoperative sagittal T2WI MRI section shows a tethered cord with a low-lying conus ending at the L4-5 level and a dorsal dermal sinus. **(b)** Postoperative sagittal T2WI MRI and **(c)** postgadolinium T1WI fat-suppressed image show a rim-enhancing intramedullary abscess with proximal cord edema and a subcutaneous abscess at the operative site.

However, treatment may be extended or altered based on the response.

Radiographic features of healing include progressive sclerosis with fusion of the affected vertebral bodies. Despite the healing of the lesion, deformity at the affected site may be seen, depending on the part of the spinal column involved and the amount of vertebra lost initially (**Fig. 3.2c,d**). MRI findings indicative of a healing response are resolution of marrow edema, fatty replacement of marrow, and resolution of cord signal changes and paravertebral/ epidural abscess (**Fig. 3.14**).[46] The MRI evidence of healing lags behind clinical improvement by about 2 months. In the follow-up MRI, it is not uncommon to note the presence of persistent changes or even a flare-up in the initial few months of treatment.[47] Hence, MRI as a tool of assessment of healing response must be used cautiously, preferably after 4 months.

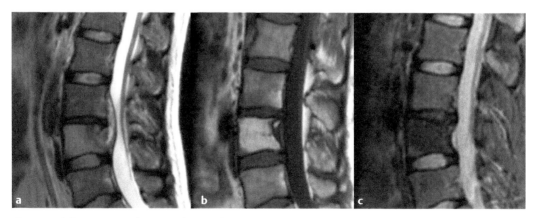

Fig. 3.14 **(a)** T2WI sagittal section shows tuberculosis spondylitis in the L4 vertebral body with marrow edema and L3–4 anterior epidural abscess. **(b)** T1WI and **(c)** T2 short tau inversion recovery (STIR) sagittal sections show fatty marrow replacement, with no residual marrow edema and complete resolution of the epidural abscess.

However, if MRI shows a deteriorating picture beyond 5 to 6 months of treatment, we should suspect a therapeutically refractory case.

Other Rare Infections

Brucella Vertebral Osteomyelitis

It is often difficult to diagnose and differentiate brucellosis from TB. Brucellosis has a predilection for the lower lumbar spine, and facet joint involvement is not uncommon. It can be of either focal or diffuse involvement.[48] The vertebral architecture is maintained despite evidence of diffuse pan-vertebral involvement (**Fig. 3.15**). Gas within the disk, smaller paraspinal abscesses, and, rarely, gibbus deformity and development of large "carrot beak" osteophytes can also be seen.

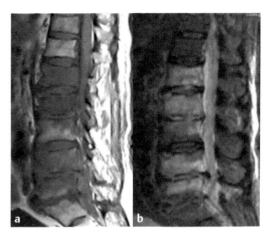

Fig. 3.15 (a) A STIR sequence and **(b)** T1WI in a case of *Brucella* spondylitis demonstrate marrow edema with preserved vertebral height of involved lumbar vertebral bodies, reduced disk heights, and end-plate erosions.

Fungal Spondylodiskitis

Imaging characteristics can be similar to those of TB, with relative sparing of the disk and anterior body involvement. Multiple vertebral levels can be involved in aspergillosis (**Fig. 3.16**),[49] blastomycosis, and candidal infections.[50] A high index of suspicion for fungal infections should be raised in immunocompromised individuals. Biopsy is essential to confirm the diagnosis.

Hydatid Disease of Spine

Hydatid disease shows early soft tissue involvement and late bony changes. Multiple cystic fluid-filled lesions with thin walls and irregular branching resembling a grape bunch may be seen on MRI at multiple levels, involving the vertebrae and the epidural and intradural regions.[51]

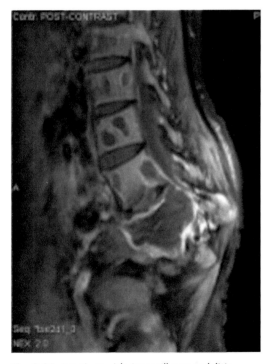

Fig. 3.16 A patient with *Aspergillus* spondylitis showing kyphotic deformity, destruction, collapse of the lower lumbar vertebrae, marrow enhancement of the upper lumbar vertebrae, with non-enhancing hypointense intraosseous abscesses.

Differential Diagnosis

A limitation of imaging is that it demonstrates the presence of several nonspecific imaging findings that may look similar to, and even

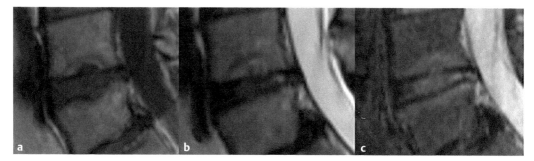

Fig. 3.17 Modic type I end-plate changes: **(a)** smooth subchondral sharp crescentic margins, with hypointense signal on T1WI; **(b)** isointense on T2WI; and **(c)** hyperintense on fat-suppressed STIR sagittal sections.

mimic, noninfective disorders. The following points can be useful to differentiate these findings from infective spondylodiskitis:

Modic Type I End-Plate Change

The Modic type I end-plate change shows a crescentic smooth subchondral marrow abnormality with an intact cortical end-plate and layering effect (**Fig. 3.17a**). In controversial cases, follow-up MRI is recommended to assess the progression. A special diffusion-weighted sequence may be helpful in differentiating degenerative changes from infectious subchondral edema, which can show the claw sign.[52] Well-defined linear demarcation is seen between normal and abnormal marrow in the Modic type I degenerative change, but not in infectious disease.

Neuropathic Spondyloarthropathy

Neuropathic spondyloarthropathy can be due to sequelae of cord injury, syrinx, or diabetes mellitus. It can demonstrate disk space loss with marginal osteophytes, the vacuum phenomenon in the disk (**Fig. 3.18c**), facet disorganization with effusion, distention and debris, and associated spondylolisthesis.[53]

Malignancy

Isolated collapse of the vertebral body with marrow signal alteration can be seen in both

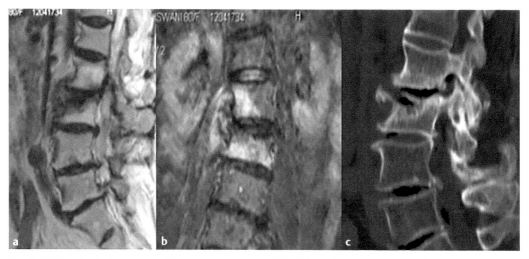

Fig. 3.18 A patient with neuropathic spondyloarthropathy showing salient features: **(a)** extensive subchondral marrow edema on T2 sagittal section, **(b)** left lateral scoliosis in coronal MRI STIR image, and **(c)** the presence of a multiple-level vacuum phenomenon in a CT sagittal section.

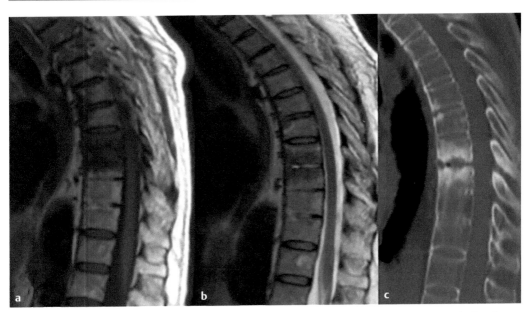

Fig. 3.19 Andersson's lesion in ankylosing spondylitis. **(a,b)** Sagittal T1WI and T2WI MRI scans show inflammatory diskovertebral destruction and subchondral marrow changes. **(c)** Bamboo spine appearance with syndesmophytes, marked endplate erosion, and subchondral marrow sclerosis are seen best on a CT reconstructed sagittal section.

TB and malignancy. In malignancy there is a usual relative sparing of disk and lack of soft tissue abscess. Sparing of the neural arch and involvement of the disk favors TB. "Good disk, bad news; bad disk, good news" is a useful phrase to remember. However, atypical skip lesions of TB may resemble neoplasm.[54]

Sarcoidosis

Sarcoidosis is a chronic inflammatory lesion characterized by noncaseating granulomas, and it may produce multifocal lesions of the vertebrae and disks, along with the meninges and paraspinal masses that appear identical to tuberculosis.[55]

Andersson's Lesion in Ankylosing Spondylitis

Andersson's lesion in ankylosing spondylitis refers to the diskovertebral lesions either secondary to inflammation or owing to stress fracture and mechanical failure, resulting in pseudarthrosis. Plain radiography does not show these lesions often. MRI shows irregular signal intensity changes (**Fig. 3.19**), thus mimicking early stages of infection, but the lesion lacks soft tissue involvement and abscess formation, and CT (**Fig. 3.19c**) often demonstrates sclerotic changes on either side of these lesions, along with the characteristic bamboo spine appearance associated with syndesmophytes formation.[56]

▣ Chapter Summary

Advances in imaging techniques have resulted in early diagnosis of spinal infections. MRI is the gold standard imaging investigation of choice in infection. However, it is not specific enough to determine the subtype of the infection, and MRI alone cannot be proposed as a single diagnostic tool. Contrast-enhanced MRI provides further detail and helps in differentiating other clinical conditions. Clinical and laboratory parameter correlation with imaging is essential to treat spinal infections appropriately. Although a CT scan helps in surgical planning, it is not essential in all cases. Nuclear scans are not only expensive but also highly nonspecific, and hence are used only in doubtful scenarios. For routine follow-up, radiography is adequate. There is an increasing trend toward the use of MRI for assessing treatment response.

Pearls

- ◆ Spinal infections need to be diagnosed early to initiate prompt treatment and to avoid irreversible neurologic injury or permanent damage to the structures that provide stability to the spine. Advanced imaging techniques aid in achieving the earliest diagnosis.
- ◆ MRI is the imaging technique that demonstrates infection earliest, in the form of bone marrow signal intensity changes, and it has the ability to detect satellite and skip lesions of spinal infections.
- ◆ MRI, and especially contrast-enhanced MRI, has the potential to differentiate tuberculosis and pyogenic infections. In addition, MRI can differentiate spinal infections from other pathological conditions of the spine such as degeneration, inflammation, and malignancy.

- ◆ MRI is the gold standard imaging of choice to assess intraspinal involvement.
- ◆ CT helps in detecting the extent of osseous destruction, thereby assessing the stability of the spine. Thus, it aids the surgeon in determining the modality of surgical intervention.
- ◆ Imaging-guided diagnostic and therapeutic procedures increase the accuracy of the procedure.
- ◆ Follow-up MRI helps in assessing the response to treatment, and therefore allows the surgeon to extend the duration of or alter the treatment whenever needed.

Pitfalls

- ◆ A radiograph can be deceptively normal in the initial stages of the infection.
- ◆ CT scan gives limited information regarding the contents of the spinal canal.
- ◆ MRI is challenging in postoperative cases with implant due to magnetic susceptibility artifacts.
- ◆ MRI is absolutely contraindicated in patients with cardiac pacemakers, cochlear implants, or other metal foreign bodies.
- ◆ Scintigraphy can show false-positive results.

References
Five Must-Read References

1. Kourbeti IS, Tsiodras S, Boumpas DT. Spinal infections: evolving concepts. Curr Opin Rheumatol 2008; 20:471–479
2. Duarte RM, Vaccaro AR. Spinal infection: state of the art and management algorithm. Eur Spine J 2013;22: 2787–2799
3. Ledermann HP, Schweitzer ME, Morrison WB, Carrino JA. MR imaging findings in spinal infections: rules or myths? Radiology 2003;228:506–514
4. Gouliouris T, Aliyu SH, Brown NM. Spondylodiscitis: update on diagnosis and management. J Antimicrob Chemother 2010;65(suppl 3):iii11–iii24
5. An HS, Seldomridge JA. Spinal infections: diagnostic tests and imaging studies. Clin Orthop Relat Res 2006;444:27–33
6. Bhavan KP, Marschall J, Olsen MA, Fraser VJ, Wright NM, Warren DK. The epidemiology of hematogenous vertebral osteomyelitis: a cohort study in a tertiary care hospital. BMC Infect Dis 2010;10:158
7. Jevtic V. Vertebral infection. Eur Radiol 2004;14(3, Suppl 3)E43–E52
8. Sapico FL, Montgomerie JZ. Pyogenic vertebral osteomyelitis: report of nine cases and review of the literature. Rev Infect Dis 1979;1:754–776
9. Varma R, Lander P, Assaf A. Imaging of pyogenic infectious spondylodiskitis. Radiol Clin North Am 2001;39:203–213
10. Jain A. Tuberculosis of the spine. Bone Joint J 2010; 92:905–913
11. DeSanto J, Ross JS. Spine infection/inflammation. Radiol Clin North Am 2011;49:105–127
12. Tali ET. Spinal infections. Eur J Radiol 2004;50:120–133
13. Khurjekar KS, Khurjekar DK, Kanikdaley VP, Shyam A. Imaging in spinal infections. Spinal Infect Trauma 2011;25
14. Ross JS, Moore KR. Diagnostic Imaging: Spine E-Book. New York: Elsevier Health Sciences; 2015
15. Veena C, Kumar GA, Niranjan K. Diagnostic Radiology: Musculoskeletal and Breast Imaging. New Delhi: Jaypee Brothers Medical Publishers; 2012
16. Acosta FL Jr, Galvez LF, Aryan HE, Ames CP. Recent advances: infections of the spine. Curr Infect Dis Rep 2006;8:390–393
17. Weinstein MA, McCabe JP, Cammisa FP Jr. Postoperative spinal wound infection: a review of 2,391 consecutive index procedures. J Spinal Disord 2000;13: 422–426

18. Mylona E, Samarkos M, Kakalou E, Fanourgiakis P, Skoutelis A. Pyogenic vertebral osteomyelitis: a systematic review of clinical characteristics. Semin Arthritis Rheum 2009;39:10–17

19. Rivas-Garcia A, Sarria-Estrada S, Torrents-Odin C, Casas-Gomila L, Franquet E. Imaging findings of Pott's disease. Eur Spine J 2013;22(4, Suppl 4)567–578

20. Chapman M, Murray RO, Stoker DJ. Tuberculosis of the bones and joints. Semin Roentgenol 1979;14:266–282

21. Tuli SM, Srivastava TP, Varma BP, Sinha GP. Tuberculosis of spine. Acta Orthop Scand 1967;38:445–458

22. Whelan MA, Schonfeld S, Post JD, et al. Computed tomography of nontuberculous spinal infection. J Comput Assist Tomogr 1985;9:280–287

23. Jain R, Sawhney S, Berry M. Computed tomography of vertebral tuberculosis: patterns of bone destruction. Clin Radiol 1993;47:196–199

24. Diehn FE. Imaging of spine infection. Radiol Clin North Am 2012;50:777–798

25. Acharya J, Gibbs WN. Imaging spinal infection. Radiol Infect Dis 2016;3:84–91

26. Lee KY. Comparison of pyogenic spondylitis and tuberculous spondylitis. Asian Spine J 2014;8:216–223

27. Jung N-Y, Jee W-H, Ha K-Y, Park C-K, Byun J-Y. Discrimination of tuberculous spondylitis from pyogenic spondylitis on MRI. AJR Am J Roentgenol 2004;182:1405–1410

28. Park JH, Shin HS, Park JT, Kim TY, Eom KS. Differentiation between tuberculous spondylitis and pyogenic spondylitis on MR imaging. Korean J Spine 2011;8:283–287

29. Murphy KJ, Brunberg JA, Quint DJ, Kazanjian PH. Spinal cord infection: myelitis and abscess formation. AJNR Am J Neuroradiol 1998;19:341–348

30. Hetem SF, Schils JP. Imaging of infections and inflammatory conditions of the spine. Semin Musculoskelet Radiol 2000;4:329–347

31. Uchida K, Nakajima H, Yayama T, et al. Epidural abscess associated with pyogenic spondylodiscitis of the lumbar spine; evaluation of a new MRI staging classification and imaging findings as indicators of surgical management: a retrospective study of 37 patients. Arch Orthop Trauma Surg 2010;130:111–118

32. Redfern RM, Miles J, Banks AJ, Dervin E. Stabilisation of the infected spine. J Neurol Neurosurg Psychiatry 1988;51:803–807

33. Skendros P, Kamaria F, Kontopoulos V, Tsitouridis I, Sidiropoulos L. Intradural, extramedullary tuberculoma of the spinal cord as a complication of tuberculous meningitis. Infection 2003;31:115–117

34. Ross JS, Masaryk TJ, Modic MT, et al. MR imaging of lumbar arachnoiditis. AJR Am J Roentgenol 1987;149:1025–1032

35. Gemmel F, Dumarey N, Palestro CJ. Radionuclide imaging of spinal infections. Eur J Nucl Med Mol Imaging 2006;33:1226–1237

36. Corstens FH, van der Meer JW. Nuclear medicine's role in infection and inflammation. In: Lancet 1999; 28(354):765–770 New York: Elsevier; 1999

37. Gratz S, Dörner J, Fischer U, et al. 18F-FDG hybrid PET in patients with suspected spondylitis. Eur J Nucl Med Mol Imaging 2002;29:516–524

38. Zhuang H, Pourdehnad M, Lambright ES, et al. Dual time point 18F-FDG PET imaging for differentiating malignant from inflammatory processes. J Nucl Med 2001;42:1412–1417

39. Tian M, Zhang H, Oriuchi N, Higuchi T, Endo K. Comparison of 11C-choline PET and FDG PET for the differential diagnosis of malignant tumors. Eur J Nucl Med Mol Imaging 2004;31:1064–1072

40. Gallucci PM, D'Orazio F. Image guided interventions in spinal infections. Neuroimaging Clin N Am 2015; 25:281–294

41. Chew FS, Kline MJ. Diagnostic yield of CT-guided percutaneous aspiration procedures in suspected spontaneous infectious diskitis. Radiology 2001;218:211–214

42. Gupta S, Suri S, Gulati M, Singh P. Ilio-psoas abscesses: percutaneous drainage under image guidance. Clin Radiol 1997;52:704–707

43. Boden SD, Davis DO, Dina TS, Sunner JL, Wiesel SW. Postoperative diskitis: distinguishing early MR imaging findings from normal postoperative disk space changes. Radiology 1992;184:765–771

44. Nouh MR. Spinal fusion-hardware construct: basic concepts and imaging review. World J Radiol 2012; 4:193–207

45. Grane P, Josephsson A, Seferlis A, Tullberg T. Septic and aseptic post-operative discitis in the lumbar spine—evaluation by MR imaging. Acta Radiol 1998; 39:108–115

46. Wang Q, Babyn P, Branson H, Tran D, Davila J, Mueller EL. Utility of MRI in the follow-up of pyogenic spinal infection in children. Pediatr Radiol 2010;40:118–130

47. Hong SH, Choi J-Y, Lee JW, Kim NR, Choi J-A, Kang HS. MR imaging assessment of the spine: infection or an imitation? Radiographics 2009;29:599–612

48. Colmenero JD, Cisneros JM, Orjuela DL, et al. Clinical course and prognosis of Brucella spondylitis. Infection 1992;20:38–42

49. Mawk JR, Erickson DL, Chou SN, Seljeskog EL. Aspergillus infections of the lumbar disc spaces. Report of three cases. J Neurosurg 1983;58:270–274

50. Palmisano A, Benecchi M, De Filippo M, Maggiore U, Buzio C, Vaglio A. Candida sake as the causative agent of spondylodiscitis in a hemodialysis patient. Spine J 2011;11:e12–e16

51. Işlekel S, Erşahin Y, Zileli M, et al. Spinal hydatid disease. Spinal Cord 1998;36:166–170

52. Patel KB, Poplawski MM, Pawha PS, Naidich TP, Tanenbaum LN. Diffusion-weighted MRI "claw sign" improves differentiation of infectious from degenerative Modic type 1 signal changes of the spine. AJNR Am J Neuroradiol 2014;35:1647–1652

53. Rothschild BM, Behnam S. The often overlooked digital tuft: clues to diagnosis and pathophysiology of neuropathic disease and spondyloarthropathy. Ann Rheum Dis 2005;64:286–290

54. Sivalingam J, Kumar A. Spinal tuberculosis resembling neoplastic lesions on MRI. J Clin Diagn Res 2015;9:TC01–TC03

55. Rúa-Figueroa I, Gantes MA, Erausquin C, Mhaidli H, Montesdeoca A. Vertebral sarcoidosis: clinical and imaging findings. Semin Arthritis Rheum 2002;31: 346–352

56. Rasker JJ, Prevo RL, Lanting PJ. Spondylodiscitis in ankylosing spondylitis, inflammation or trauma? A description of six cases. Scand J Rheumatol 1996; 25:52–57

4

Instrumentation and Spinal Infections

Hisam Muhamad Ariffin, Yoshiharu Kawaguchi, and ChungChek Wong

Introduction

The use of spinal instrumentation is on the rise. Various instrumentation systems have been developed in an effort to manage a myriad of spinal pathologies and trauma, and to perform deformity correction, stabilization, and fusion of the spinal column. These instrumentation systems take different forms and serve different biomechanical functions. Constructs such as pedicle screws and rods, plates and screws or hooks, and sublaminar wiring provide stability, whereas titanium mesh, expandable cages, and polyetheretherketone (PEEK) interbody fusion cages lend structural support. Artificial disks are the most complex form of spinal instrumentation in terms of their material composition and their multiple interfaces. Though various spinal instrumentation systems have helped patients achieve structural support and stability, difficulties arise when spinal infections occur.

We may classify infection of the spine, based on the site of infection, as spondylodiskitis, diskitis, epidural abscess, septic facet arthropathy, and vertebral body involvement. These entities are not mutually exclusive, and patients may present with infection at several sites. Not uncommonly, the spinal column is rendered unstable, resulting in pain, deformity, and possibly neurologic insult when significant bony destruction has occurred.

The discussion of instrumentation and spine infection can entail two clinical scenarios, namely the use of instrumentation in the vicinity of active de novo spine infection, and the use of spine instrumentation and its associated potential consequence of surgical site infection. The discussion about infection typically revolves around whether the causative organism is of tuberculous origin or is a pyogenic organism. With regard to implant retention versus implant removal in the presence of postoperative surgical site infection, there are many important clinical issues to be addressed. New research on the use of implants in the presence of active spinal infection will help improve the management of these patients.

The response of the human body to an implant is still not fully understood, and the interaction of the microorganism with both the material and the host adds another layer of complexity.

Relationship Among Implants, Host, and Microorganisms

The presence of foreign material in the human body is known to elicit a host response. Once foreign material is implanted in the body, a layer of plasma proteins, such as fibrinogen, albumin, and fibronectin, coats the material's surface, leading to acute inflammation. The inflammation then becomes chronic, and a fibrous encapsulation of the material occurs as a result of a foreign body reaction. This fibrous capsule, being relatively avascular, confers limited access to both systemic antibiotics and the host immune defense.

The inception of biomaterial-associated infection begins with the colonization of an implant surface with bacteria, which can occur both perioperatively in the operating room as well as postoperatively as a consequence of hematogenous seeding. The race for the implant surface between the microorganism and the host immune defense commences immediately following implant placement within an area of active infection intraoperatively. In the case of postoperative contamination that occurs after spinal instrumentation, the microorganism may adhere to the protein molecules on the implant surface, forming a biofilm that is resistant to antibiotics.

The affinity of bacteria for any surface is affected by the material's topography, especially its surface roughness, and the material's surface chemistry, notably the wettability.[1]

The study of surface affinity of bacteria is strain specific, because the strain's physical size, surface topography, and adhesion molecules vary. The presence of protein molecules in vivo also significantly alters bacteria adhesion to the material.

One strategy to reduce bacteria adherence to biofilm is to coat the PEEK implant with titanium dioxide and polydimethylsiloxane (PDMS), which enables the regulated release of antimicrobial silver. The hybrid coating also inhibits bacterial growth and biofilm formation.

Asymptomatic bacteria colonization of the cervical plate used in the treatment of vertebral osteomyelitis has been documented in patients whose implants were removed after healing of the infection.[2] However, these patients did not exhibit active ongoing infection of the spine. It appears that the presence of microorganisms in the biofilm can be limited to only the implant surface, avoiding the adjacent tissue environment.

Thus, the fibrous capsule that renders the area relatively avascular is formed only on the implant (pedicle screw and rods) surface and does not surround the entire area of infection. Since the biofilm is formed only around the implants, an adjacent focus of osteomyelitis with adequate blood supply can progress to healing, unaffected by the implant biofilm. Infection of the artificial disk replacement, on the other hand, poses a different problem, as the focus of infection is encased within the fibrous capsule itself.

Postoperative Infection Following Spinal Instrumentation Surgery

Infection following spinal instrumentation surgeries differs from instrumentation in the presence of de novo spinal infection, in several ways. The causative microorganism in the former scenario, since it is hospital-acquired, commonly involves multiresistant strains, such as the methicillin-resistant *Staphylococcus aureus*, or opportunistic microorganisms, such as *Staphylococcus epidermidis* or fungal infection. As well, the host in the former scenario patients generally are healthier than patients with a pyogenic spinal infection.

Spine surgery with instrumentation is associated with a higher risk of surgical site infection than is spine surgery without instrumentation, for several reasons. Spinal instrumentation surgeries tend to be more complex than noninstrumented spine surgeries, involving longer operating time, more soft tissue injury, greater blood loss, and more operating room personnel. The presence of foreign materials in the surgical site may dampen the host defense mechanisms. As well, the physical presence of hooks, pedicle screws, and rods in posterior spine surgery increases the dead space in the surgical wound and could thus predispose to surgical site infection.

Diagnosis of a spine surgical site infection may be challenging at times. The classical signs of increasing wound pain, wound edge redness, wound discharge, and systemic effects of infection may be absent. Laboratory results may be equivocal, making it difficult for clinicians to differentiate between postoperative wound inflammation and surgical site infection.

Imaging modality utilization in cases of suspected surgical site infection with implantation can be an arduous undertaking. In chronic infection with bony erosion, a plain computed tomography (CT) scan may be diagnostic. In early surgical site infection, however, imaging may not be very helpful. Although magnetic resonance imaging (MRI) has been used to detect early peri-implant osteomyelitis or intervertebral abscess, imaging artifacts from the implants coupled with postoperative inflammatory changes often complicate making a diagnosis, further defeating the value of imaging in the detection of early spine surgical site infection. Recently, ^{18}F-fluorodeoxyglucose (FDG) positron emission tomography (PET) scanning has been advocated as the imaging most likely to confirm the presence of infection in the instrumented spine.[3]

The general algorithm for treatment depends on a variety of factors, including the time delay from the index procedure, the infecting microorganism, the location and extent of the infection, the strength of the fusion mass, and the stability of the spine prior to the instrumentation.

Retention of spinal instrumentation or implant exchange following wound debridement for postoperative surgical site infections is generally attempted in patients who presented within 3 months of the index surgery,[4] because the intended fusion has yet to take place. However, the continued presence of instrumentation in these patients predisposes them to recurrent infection. Repeated wound debridement or prolonged wound suction drainage (open or closed) may thus be necessary to treat patients with recurrent infection.[5]

Removal of instrumentation after surgical site infection of spine surgery is called for when the infection persists despite repeated serial debridement.

Late-onset surgical site infection is usually treated with wound debridement and removal of the implant because fusion has taken place. There may be possible progression of spinal deformity after removal of the implant in patients whose spine has already solidly fused.

Instrumentation in Tuberculous Infection of the Spine

After it was discovered that *Mycobacterium tuberculosis* cannot form a biofilm on the implant, as compared with a pyogenic microorganism,[6] various types of implant (stainless steel, titanium, and PEEK), including anterior interbody fusion cages and pedicle screws, have been used to treat spinal tuberculosis in order to correct the deformity, achieve spinal stabilization, and enable early mobilization of these patients.

Recently, posterior instrumentation of the spine with tuberculous infection without debridement was shown to be an effective treatment, demonstrated by the eradication of infection and solid fusion of the anterior column (tuberculous spondylodiskitis foci).[7] This suggests that stabilization of the spine leads to higher fusion rates and healing of the lesions. Posterior instrumentation of the spine in this regard would have to involve multiple segments so that it can provide adequate cantilever support to the deficient anterior column until solid fusion takes place.

Instrumentation in Active Pyogenic Infection of the Spine

Spinal instrumentation in the presence of active spinal infection has been viewed as a high-risk practice, presumably as a consequence of the experiences derived from orthopedic surgery, particularly arthroplasty surgery. A two-stage procedure is the standard practice. The first stage entails debriding the infected site. The second stage, which is performed after allowing

Table 4.1 Posterior Single-Stage Debridement and Instrumentation Studies

Author (Year)	Number of Patients	Number of Recurrences	Fusion Rate (%)	Lost to Follow-Up
Kim and Choi[8] (2016)	33	0	100	0
Lu et al[9] (2015)	28	3	82	0
Mohamed et al[10] (2014)	15	0	–	0
Tschöke et al[11] (2015)	18	0	100	0
Lee and Suh[12] (2006)	18	0	100	0
Shetty et al[13] (2016)	27	0	100	0
Lin et al[14] (2012)	48	0	–	0
Gorensek et al[15] (2013)	17	0	88	0
An et al[16] (2012)	15	0	100	0
Lee et al[17] (2014)	10	0	100	0

sufficient time for the infection to be eradicated, entails implantation of the prosthesis. Unfortunately, by avoiding instrumentation in pyogenic spondylodiskitis, patients are inevitably being subjected to persistent pain, prolonged bed rest, lengthy hospitalization, and residual deformity of the spine.

In the event that spinal instrumentation is deemed necessary, various surgical approaches and strategies have been employed for the treatment of pyogenic spondylodiskitis. Because most spine pyogenic infection involves the anterior column, anterior debridement followed by autologous bone graft is the de facto judicious practice. Autologous bone graft, although initially avascular, is held to be resistant to infection as it is not a foreign material. In circumstances where immediate stability is necessary, posterior instrumentation is proposed to avoid contamination of the implant from the site of active infection.

Among the many surgical approaches, the single-stage posterior transforaminal or transpedicular approach to debride the infection focus followed by posterior pedicle screw stabilization would hypothetically confer the greatest likelihood of implant contamination, because the implant is in direct continuity with the foci of spondylodiskitis. Furthermore, the debridement process is limited to posterior access alone, potentially leaving loads of residual microorganisms. In this regard, bacteria adherence to the implant surface and hence

biofilm production will again hypothetically lead to persistence of the infection postoperatively. **Table 4.1** summarizes 10 such studies reported in the literatures. Nine of the 10 retrospective studies, involving a total of 201 patients, found no recurrence or persistence of the spondylodiskitis after surgery. The remaining study reported that three of 28 patients experienced recurrence of infection. These studies suggest that the use of pedicle screw stabilization is in fact safe in the presence of active infection of the spine. Likewise, many studies also demonstrated similar result with the use of titanium mesh and PEEK cages in spondylodiskitis.

Several hypotheses were postulated by the authors who reported success with the single-stage posterior transformational or transpedicular debridement followed by the posterior stabilization technique. One author supplemented this technique with prolonged wound suction drainage for an average of 16 days.[8] The feasibility of this strategy was attributed to the elimination of potential dead space (which provides an inherent fertile ground for bacteria multiplication) by the use of suction drains. Another author postulated that stabilization with instrumentation of the spine helped in the host defense against the infective organism.[18] Also, as described earlier, pedicle screws and rods do not form biofilm surrounding the entire area of infection; therefore, systemic administration of antibiotics and local host defense mechanisms could still be active against the infective organism.

Thus, it appears from these recent studies that spinal instrumentation in the presence of active spinal infection is a safe practice.[19] It does not present a difficulty in infection eradication. Some authors even suggested that spinal stabilization with instrumentation improves the outcome.[20] Proposed benefits include accelerated granulation tissue growth and soft tissue healing. Two studies demonstrated that posterior pedicle screw stabilization without debridement of the infection foci leads to healing and fusion of the spondylodiskitis.

Findings from several studies do not show significant differences in infection recurrence rates between treatment with antibiotic therapy alone, antibiotic therapy and surgical debridement with autologous bone grafting, and antibiotic therapy with spinal instrumentation.

If implant utilization in spondylodiskitis is safe as shown in the various recent retrospective studies, perhaps its advocated use should be more widespread so that patients can be mobilized early, as there are strong indications that early mobilization can lead to better patient survival from spinal infection by limiting bed-ridden complications such as pulmonary atelectasis, thromboembolic phenomenons, and disuse muscle atrophy. Nevertheless, the use of instrumentation in spinal infection to correct kyphotic deformity has yet to be proven clinically to improve pain.

◼ Chapter Summary

Spine instrumentation provides stability, corrects deformity, maintains alignment, and enhances fusion. Often patients with spinal infections, pyogenic or tuberculous, present with deformity and instability that may require spinal instrumentation. Implant use in these situations is shadowed by concerns that bacteria adherent to the implant surface will lead to difficulty in infection eradication. This biofilm is resistant to antibiotics and host defense mechanisms. Research showed that *M. tuberculosis* does not adhere to these surfaces as readily as pyogenic bacteria. Anterior structural support, plates and screws, posterior pedicle screw fixation with stainless steel, titanium, or PEEK have been used in tuberculous infection of the spine without evidence of persistence of the infection.

In pyogenic infection of the spine, a more prudent approach has been observed. The last decade saw many reports on the use of instrumentation in pyogenic spondylodiskitis, with encouraging results. Even in situations where the implants were used with a high possibility of contamination by the infective organism, the incidence of recurrence of infection was very low. This surprising finding could be due to the relatively minor effect of the implant biofilm on the entire spondylodiskitis milieu. Another strategy commonly employed is the reduction of potential dead space by prolonged wound suction drainage.

Surgeries on the noninfected spine with implant are associated with a higher risk of surgical site infection than spine surgeries without an implant. These infections are also more likely to require repeated wound debridement. Nonetheless, these complications could be managed most of the time with wound debridement and retention of the implant, especially in patients who present within 3 months of the index surgery. Removal of hardware is indicated in patients with persistence of infection despite repeated wound debridement, in patients with implant loosening, and in patients who have achieved fusion.

- Pedicle screws, rod, plates, interbody cages, and mesh made of stainless steel, titanium, or PEEK is safe to be used in the presence of active pyogenic and tuberculous infection of the spine.
- When biomechanical principles are adhered to, the use of posterior instrumentation of the unstable spondylodiskitis can rapidly reduce pain, correct deformity, and lead to solid fusion.
- Wound debridement and retention of the implant in the event of early surgical site infection can result in resolution of the infection, although sometimes repeated debridement or prolonged wound suction drainage may be necessary.

- Even though bacteria will form a biofilm and adhere to the surface of the spine implant, the infective foci will progress to healing and fusion, if treated adequately with appropriate antibiotics and debridement.

- An artificial disk replacement should not be implanted at the site of active infection in the spine.
- Reluctance to use spine instrumentation to stabilize the unstable spondylodiskitis for fear of recurrence of infection is inappropriate.
- Do not retain infected implants that are loosened, for loss of stability is associated with persistence of the infection.

References
Five Must-Read References

1. Rochford ET, Poulsson AH, Salavarrieta Varela J, Lezuo P, Richards RG, Moriarty TF. Bacterial adhesion to orthopaedic implant materials and a novel oxygen plasma modified PEEK surface. Colloids Surf B Biointerfaces 2014;113:213–222
2. Shad A, Shariff S, Fairbank J, Byren I, Teddy PJ, Cadoux-Hudson TA. Internal fixation for osteomyelitis of cervical spine: the issue of persistence of culture positive infection around the implants. Acta Neurochir (Wien) 2003;145:957–960, discussion 960
3. Inanami H, Oshima Y, Iwahori T, Takano Y, Koga H, Iwai H. Role of 18F-fluoro-D-deoxyglucose PET/CT in diagnosing surgical site infection after spine surgery with instrumentation. Spine 2015;40:109–113
4. Glotzbecker MP, Gomez JA, Miller PE, et al. Management of spinal implants in acute pediatric surgical site infections: a multicenter study. Spine Deform 2016;4:277–282
5. Dipaola CP, Saravanja DD, Boriani L, et al. Postoperative infection treatment score for the spine (PITSS): construction and validation of a predictive model to define need for single versus multiple irrigation and debridement for spinal surgical site infection. Spine J 2012;12:218–230
6. Ha K-Y, Chung Y-G, Ryoo S-J. Adherence and biofilm formation of Staphylococcus epidermidis and Mycobacterium tuberculosis on various spinal implants. Spine 2005;30:38–43
7. Wang ST, Ma HL, Lin CP, et al. Anterior debridement may not be necessary in the treatment of tuberculous spondylitis of the thoracic and lumbar spine in adults: a retrospective study. Bone Joint J 2016;98-B: 834–839
8. Kim YM, Choi SM. Posterior only approach for lumbar pyogenic spondylitis with short instrumentation and prolonged suction drainage. Spine 2016;41:E1022–E1029
9. Lu ML, Niu CC, Tsai TT, Fu TS, Chen LH, Chen WJ. Transforaminal lumbar interbody debridement and fusion for the treatment of infective spondylodiscitis in the lumbar spine. Eur Spine J 2015;24:555–560
10. Mohamed AS, Yoo J, Hart R, et al. Posterior fixation without debridement for vertebral body osteomyelitis and discitis. Neurosurg Focus 2014;37:E6
11. Tschöke SK, Fuchs H, Schmidt O, Gulow J, von der Hoeh NH, Heyde CE. Single-stage debridement and spinal fusion using PEEK cages through a posterior approach for eradication of lumbar pyogenic spondylodiscitis: a safe treatment strategy for a detrimental condition. Patient Saf Surg 2015;9:35
12. Lee JS, Suh KT. Posterior lumbar interbody fusion with an autogenous iliac crest bone graft in the treatment of pyogenic spondylodiscitis. J Bone Joint Surg Br 2006;88:765–770
13. Shetty AP, Aiyer SN, Kanna RM, Maheswaran A, Rajasekaran S. Pyogenic lumbar spondylodiscitis treated with transforaminal lumbar interbody fusion: safety and outcomes. Int Orthop 2016;40:1163–1170
14. Lin CP, Ma HL, Wang ST, Liu CL, Yu WK, Chang MC. Surgical results of long posterior fixation with short fusion in the treatment of pyogenic spondylodiscitis of the thoracic and lumbar spine: a retrospective study. Spine 2012;37:E1572–E1579
15. Gorensek M, Kosak R, Travnik L, Vengust R. Posterior instrumentation, anterior column reconstruction with single posterior approach for treatment of pyo-

genic osteomyelitis of thoracic and lumbar spine. Eur Spine J 2013;22:633–641

16. An KC, Kim JY, Kim TH, et al. Posterior lumbar interbody fusion using compressive bone graft with allograft and autograft in the pyogenic discitis. Asian Spine J 2012;6:15–21

17. Lee BH, Park JO, Kim HS, Lee HM, Cho BW, Moon SH. Transpedicular curettage and drainage versus combined anterior and posterior surgery in infectious spondylodiscitis. Indian J Orthop 2014;48:74–80

18. Rayes M, Colen CB, Bahgat DA, et al. Safety of instrumentation in patients with spinal infection. J Neurosurg Spine 2010;12:647–659

19. Dennis Hey HW, Nathaniel Ng LW, Tan CS, et al. Spinal implants can be inserted in patients with deep spine infection: results from a large cohort study. Spine 2017;42:E490–E495

20. Dobran M, Iacoangeli M, Nasi D, et al. Posterior titanium screw fixation without debridement of infected tissue for the treatment of thoracolumbar spontaneous pyogenic spondylodiscitis. Asian Spine J 2016; 10:465–471

5

Pyogenic Spondylodiskitis: Pathogenesis and Clinical Features

Mauro Antonio Fernandes, Luiz Roberto Vialle, and Phelipe de Souza Menegaz

Introduction

Spinal infections may be classified as mycobacterial, fungal, or pyogenic.[1] Tuberculous spondylitis was once the most common form of spinal infection, but its incidence has fallen for the past 50 years due to successful diagnosis and treatment of pulmonary tuberculosis. Fungal infections are rare conditions and mainly affect immunocompromised patients. Nowadays, most cases are monomicrobial, and *Staphylococcus aureus* is the dominant organism (30–80%). Understanding the vascular anatomy of the spine, the anatomic differences between the child and adult, and the clinical presentation of pyogenic infections should assist accurate diagnosis and early treatment, avoiding serious complications.[1,2]

Pathogenesis

Spinal infections account for 2 to 7% of orthopedic infections.[3] There are three main routes for pathogen dissemination in pyogenic spondylodiskitis: hematogenous spread, contiguous spread, and direct inoculation. The hematogenous spread of bacteria is responsible for most cases of spinal infections, frequently affecting the lumbar spine in up to 58% of cases, followed by the thoracic spine in 30% of patients and the cervical spine in 11% of patients.[4] Contiguous spread occurs when bacteria spread from a contiguous focus of infection (e.g., retropharyngeal abscess and aortic implant infections). Direct inoculation often occurs as postoperative infections (e.g., after diskectomy or instrumented fusions).[5,6]

Vascular Anatomy of the Spine

In an attempt to elucidate the pathogenic pathways of vertebral infection, Batson[7] in 1940 and Wiley and Trueta[8] in 1959 described a paravertebral plexus of veins and arterial anastomoses in the vertebral body, respectively. In 1926, while studying the diploic veins in the cranial bone, Batson turned to Breschet's[9] 1828 work on the paravertebral venous plexus and its communication with the intracranial venous system. Breschet identified a longitudinal large-capacitance vertebral venous plexus, which connected to the venae cave and extended to the cranial venous sinuses. According to Breschet's study and the reports of pathologists on metastatic spread through veins, Batson believed in a connection between the vertebral venous plexus and pelvic venous system that justified bone metastases from prostate cancer. Finally, Batson reported a paravertebral plexus of veins that extended from the skull to the sacrum, which connected veins to the pelvic venous system. Changes in intra-abdominal pressure resulted in retrograde flow between these systems during physiological processes, such as coughing or straining. Therefore, it has been suggested that there is a relationship between Batson's plexus and dissemination of tumoral emboli and infections.[7,10]

Wiley and Trueta highlighted a rich arterial anastomotic system that supplied the vertebral metaphysis with terminal arterioles. Spinal arteries enter the spinal canal through the intervertebral foramen at the disk level. Ascending and descending branches supply the vertebral bodies above and below through the posterior nutrient foramina. The authors reported that the metaphyseal arterioles were more easily filled by contrast than was the venous system described by Batson. They suggested that there are two different routes of hematogenous spread: the nutrient arteries, which are easier to access by contrast injection, and the paravertebral plexus of veins, which is more difficult to fill with contrast and, therefore, is a less common dissemination route.[8]

The vascular anatomy of the spine and the anatomic differences between the child and adult explain the findings on imaging studies and clinical evaluation. In the child, the blood supply of the intervertebral disk comes from the vessels crossing the vertebral end plates and reaching the disk space. Thus, a septic embolus should cause not a bone infarction but rather an infection of the disk.[4] After 8 years of age, these vessels obliterate and the adult disk becomes avascular. At this point, disk cells depend on diffusion from the richly vascularized vertebral end plate for nutrition.[1,11] As septic emboli reach the end arterioles of the vertebral metaphysis, a suppurative inflammation begins. Initially, vascular dilatation and fluid extravasation from fenestrated vessels cause edema in the bone marrow. The pressure in the intertrabecular space increases, diminishing the local blood flow and initiating an ischemic cascade. As a result of ischemia and local suppurative process, bone necrosis occurs.[12] The disk is damaged after involvement of the vertebral end plate by enzymes, in a similar fashion to the destruction of the articular cartilage in septic arthritis. This leads to the classic spondylo-

diskitis diagnostic imaging: erosion of the vertebral end plate, osteolytic lesions, abscesses, and compression fractures that may cause spinal instability, deformity, and compression of neural elements.[4]

Occasionally, an abscess may exude through the larger sciatic notch and appear in the gluteal region, below the piriform fascia, in the perirectal region, or even in the popliteal fossa. More virulent organisms may not follow a fascial plane and may extend into the visceral structures.[11] Neurologic findings may be due to direct compression by epidural abscesses, granulation tissue, bone, or disk as spinal deformity and instability develop. In addition, the neural elements may suffer ischemic injury from septic thrombosis or inflammatory cell infiltration.[13]

Microbiology

A single organism is usually the cause of pyogenic spondylodiskitis (68%).[14,15] *Staphylococcus aureus* and *Streptococcus* species (over 50%) are the most common causative organisms, followed by gram-negative aerobic bacilli (4–30%).[16,17] Streptococci are often associated with endocarditis, *Pseudomonas* species with intravenous drug use, and *Escherichia coli* and *Proteus* species with infections of the gastrointestinal and genitourinary tract.[16,17] Anaerobic infections (3%) are frequently related to diabetes, and organisms of low virulence (coagulase negative staphylococci and streptococci viridans) to immune deficiency.[16,17] Methicillin-resistant *S. aureus* (MRSA) should be considered in endemic regions and in patients with prior infection. A polymicrobial cause is uncommon (two organisms, 21%; more than two organisms, 11%) and may be seen as a contiguous spread of infection from decubitus ulcers.[14-16]

Clinical Features

The history and clinical findings of pyogenic spondylodiskitis are determined by three major factors: the extent of the infectious process, the virulence of the causative microbial pathogen, and the host defense response.[13] Males are more commonly affected than females, with a ratio of 1.5:1 to 3:1. The age distribution is bimodal as follows: the largest group in the fifth decade and a small subset in the second decade.[1,13]

Clinical Findings in the Adult

Other sites of infection linked with hematogenous spread (e.g., genitourinary tract infection or manipulation, respiratory tract infection, skin infection), are present in up to 47% of patients. Comorbidities that predispose to spinal infection include immunosuppression, diabetes mellitus, hepatic disease, chronic kidney disease, alcoholism, and intravenous drug abuse. The two most common risk factors for pyogenic spondylodiskitis are a previous spinal procedure (39.1%) and diabetes (15.2%).[1,18]

The early findings are nonspecific, and the onset is more likely to occur gradually, which may delay the diagnosis by several months.[1] The mean time to diagnosis is 30.2 days for positive-culture cases and 72.2 days for negative-culture cases.[18] Pyogenic spondylodiskitis in intravenous drug users are most often diagnosed within 3 months (89%). Most patients with postoperative infection are diagnosed between 10 days and 2 weeks after surgery, but there have been reports of clinical presentations 2 years or longer after spinal surgery.[1] The lumbar spine is the most common location. Lesions spanning multiple levels occur in 5 to 18% of patients.[14]

The most common presenting symptom is unremitting back or neck pain, affecting ~ 90% of patients.[14] Pain is worse at night and exacerbated by movement.[1] This chief complaint is not relieved with rest, and it may radiate to the abdomen, hip, perineum, or leg.[16] Low-grade fever is present in 60 to 70% of patients.[14] Febrile episodes have been reported in 85%

of positive-culture cases and 32% of culture-negative cases.[18]

Neurologic findings are reported in 5 to 17% of cases.[1] The progression of neurologic symptoms is variable, which may be of sudden onset or follow an indolent clinical course.[19] Worsening of axial back pain, radicular signs, and paralysis may be caused by an epidural abscess or kyphotic collapse of the spine. Motor impairment is more prevalent than sensory involvement as a result of mainly anterior medullary compression.[16] Constitutional symptoms (e.g., anorexia and weight loss) may be evident.[1] Cachexia with generalized lymphadenopathy is suggestive of acquired immunodeficiency syndrome (AIDS).[1,19]

Physical examination may reveal a paravertebral muscle spasm and restriction of spinal motion.[1,19] Patients with paraspinal abscess may demonstrate hip flexion, whereas those with epidural abscess may complain of pain during straight leg raise. Painful gibbus or psoas abscess may occur in advanced disease.[19]

Diagnosing cervical pyogenic spondylodiskitis is difficult, and it may be correctly diagnosed initially in as few as 7% of patients.[20] The infection may spread anteriorly and cause retropharyngeal abscess, or inferiorly and cause mediastinitis.[19] A neurologic deficit develops in most patients (70%) due to the delay in diagnosis. The relationship between the spinal cord and the cervical spinal canal, the epidural abscess, and bone destruction are important factors in neurologic deterioration.[20]

Spinal deformity and epidural abscesses are among the main complications of pyogenic spondylodiskitis. As destruction of the vertebral body occurs, height loss may take place, leading to segmental kyphosis, whereas lateral listhesis may cause progressive scoliosis. These changes may culminate in central canal and neural foramina stenosis. Meanwhile, an epidural abscess may result in an acute neurologic deterioration. Diabetes mellitus is the most common risk factor for epidural abscess (18–54% of cases), usually affecting the lower thoracic and lumbar regions.[13]

Clinical Findings in the Child

Most spinal infections in children affect the disk space, and there is often a delay in diagnosis.[1] Scoles and Quinn[21] reported symptom duration of less than 2 weeks in 24% of patients, between 2 and 4 weeks in 38% of patients, and longer than 4 weeks in 38% of patients. Diagnosis after 4 weeks of symptoms is associated with the need for surgical treatment.[22]

History and physical findings of spondylodiskitis in the child vary with age. In general, fever is not as common as in adults, and up to 60% of patients may be afebrile.[1] In patients younger than 3 years of age, the signs and symptoms are often mild. In this group, the classic presentation is irritability (62.5%), refusal to bear weight (37.5%), limping gait (37.5%), and fever (37.5%). In patients younger than 10 years of age, the most common findings are back pain (88.8%), fever (58.8%), and abdominal pain (29.4%).[1,22]

In patients older than 10 years of age, back pain is the most prevalent symptom, and physical examination findings include localized tenderness and rigidity.[1]

Clinical Findings in the Elderly and in Postoperative Infection

The elderly population is susceptible to spinal infections due to reduced immunity; 40% of cases have subacute or chronic presentations. Diabetes mellitus is one of the main risk factors for spondylodiskitis in this age group (18–40% of patients). The incidence of paralysis is high (35–58%) and may be related to spinal canal stenosis and spinal deformity.[23]

The most common clinical presentation of the patient with postoperative infection is wound discharge and fever. The wound may be erythematous and result in dehiscence. Fever may become an important predictor of spinal infection if it persists for more than a few postoperative days.[1]

Chapter Summary

Spinal infections may be classified as mycobacterial, fungal, or pyogenic. Most cases are monomicrobial, and *S. aureus* is the dominant organism. The vascular anatomy of the spine plays a key role in the pathogenesis and clinical presentation of pyogenic spondylodiskitis. The hematogenous spread of bacteria is responsible for most cases, and the lumbar spine is the most affected region. Batson[7] and Wiley and Trueta[8] described a paravertebral plexus of veins and arterial anastomoses in the vertebral body, which are the routes of hematogenous spread. Anatomic difference between the child and adult explains the more common involvement of the intervertebral disk in younger patients.

The history and physical findings vary with age. The clinical presentation may be indolent, and the diagnosis is often delayed. Back pain and fever are the most common clinical features in adults, but early findings are usually nonspecific. The physical examination may reveal a paravertebral muscle spasm and restriction of spinal motion. Neurologic findings are reported in 5 to 17% of patients and may be caused by an epidural abscess or kyphotic collapse of the spine. Irritability is the most common symptom in patients younger than 3 years of age, and paralysis is highly prevalent in the elderly population. Spinal deformity, commonly kyphosis and epidural abscesses are among the main complications of spondylodiskitis. Prompt evaluation and accurate diagnosis may prevent severe complications.

<table>
<tr><td>

Pearls

- ◆ Hematogenous spread of bacteria through the nutrient arteries and the paravertebral plexus of veins is responsible for most cases of spinal infections.
- ◆ Back pain and fever are the most common clinical features in adults, and the lumbar spine is the most affected region.
- ◆ The clinical presentation of spondylodiskitis in the child varies with age, and fever is less common than in adults.

</td><td>

Pitfalls

- ◆ Failure to promptly evaluate and accurately diagnose pyogenic spondylodiskitis is related to the need for surgical treatment and severe complications.
- ◆ Clinical presentation is of indolent onset and nonspecific early symptoms, which may delay diagnosis.
- ◆ Progressive neurologic deficit may be caused by an epidural abscess, and it should be treated early.

</td></tr>
</table>

References

Five Must-Read References

1. Weinstein MA, Patel TC, Bell GR. Evaluation of the patient with spinal infection. Semin Spine Surg 2000; 12:60–175
2. Duarte RM, Vaccaro AR. Spinal infection: state of the art and management algorithm. Eur Spine J 2013; 22:2787–2799
3. Tyrrell PN, Cassar-Pullicino VN, McCall IW. Spinal infection. Eur Radiol 1999;9:1066–1077
4. Ratcliffe JF. Anatomic basis for the pathogenesis and radiologic features of vertebral osteomyelitis and its differentiation from childhood discitis. A microarteriographic investigation. Acta Radiol Diagn (Stockh) 1985;26:137–143
5. Silber JS, Anderson DG, Vaccaro AR, Anderson PA, McCormick P; NASS. Management of postprocedural discitis. Spine J 2002;2:279–287
6. Babinchak TJ, Riley DK, Rotheram EB Jr. Pyogenic vertebral osteomyelitis of the posterior elements. Clin Infect Dis 1997;25:221–224
7. Batson OV. The function of the vertebral veins and their role in the spread of metastases. Ann Surg 1940;112:138–149
8. Wiley AM, Trueta J. The vascular anatomy of the spine and its relationship to pyogenic vertebral osteomyelitis. J Bone Joint Surg Br 1959;41-B:796–809
9. Breschet G. Récherches Anatomiques, Physiologique et Pathologiques sur le Système Veineux et Spécialement sur les Cavaux Veineux des Os. Paris, France: Villaret et Cie; 1828–1832
10. Nathoo N, Caris EC, Wiener JA, Mendel E. History of the vertebral venous plexus and the significant contributions of Breschet and Batson. Neurosurgery 2011;69:1007–1014, discussion 1014
11. Fucs PM, Meves R, Yamada HH. Spinal infections in children: a review. Int Orthop 2012;36:387–395
12. Esendagli-Yilmaz G, Uluoglu O. Pathologic basis of pyogenic, nonpyogenic, and other spondylitis and discitis. Neuroimaging Clin N Am 2015;25:159–161
13. Arbelaez A, Restrepo F, Castillo M. Spinal infections: clinical and imaging features. Top Magn Reson Imaging 2014;23:303–314
14. Cottle L, Riordan T. Infectious spondylodiscitis. J Infect 2008;56:401–412
15. Hadjipavlou AG, Mader JT, Necessary JT, Muffoletto AJ. Hematogenous pyogenic spinal infections and their surgical management. Spine 2000;25:1668–1679
16. Skaf GS, Domloj NT, Fehlings MG, et al. Pyogenic spondylodiscitis: an overview. J Infect Public Health 2010;3:5–16
17. Cheung WY, Luk KD. Pyogenic spondylitis. Int Orthop 2012;36:397–404
18. Boody BS, Jenkins TJ, Maslak J, Hsu WK, Patel AA. Vertebral osteomyelitis and spinal epidural abscess: an evidence-based review. J Spinal Disord Tech 2015; 28:E316–E327
19. Govender S. Spinal infections. J Bone Joint Surg Br 2005;87:1454–1458
20. Miyazaki M, Yoshiiwa T, Kodera R, Tsumura H. Clinical features of cervical pyogenic spondylitis and intraspinal abscess. J Spinal Disord Tech 2011;24:E57–E61
21. Scoles PV, Quinn TP. Intervertebral discitis in children and adolescents. Clin Orthop Relat Res 1982;162: 31–36
22. Kang HM, Choi EH, Lee HJ, et al. The etiology, clinical presentation and long-term outcome of spondylodiscitis in children. Pediatr Infect Dis J 2016;35:e102–e106
23. Yoshimoto M, Takebayashi T, Kawaguchi S, et al. Pyogenic spondylitis in the elderly: a report from Japan with the most aging society. Eur Spine J 2011;20: 649–654

6

Pyogenic Spondylodiskitis: Diagnosis and Management

Joost P.H.J. Rutges, Diederik Hendrik Ruth Kempen, and F. Cumhur Oner

Introduction

The incidence of pyogenic spondylodiskitis has increased in recent decades. Whereas tuberculosis was the most important cause of spine infections during the 20th century, pyogenic spondylodiskitis is now the most common cause of primary spine infections.[1,2] Aging of the population, increased numbers of immunocompromised patients, and improved diagnostic possibilities are responsible for this increase.[1,2] As described in Chapter 5, pyogenic spondylodiskitis is one of the diagnostic challenges in modern medicine. Spondylodiskitis is a unique disease in which a diagnostic delay of up to several months is considered to be a key characteristic of the clinical presentation.[3,4] Besides the diagnostic challenges, the treatment of spondylodiskitis can be equally complex and often requires a multidisciplinary approach. Although most patients can be treated conservatively, it is important to recognize the cases in which surgical treatment is more appropriate. This chapter provides a systematic and evidence-based algorithm for the diagnosis and treatment of pyogenic spondylodiskitis.

Differential Diagnosis

Pyogenic spondylodiskitis can be difficult to diagnose and may initially be misdiagnosed due to the low frequency of the disease. Because it is often a complication of a distant infection causing bacteremia, the relatively nonspecific array of symptoms of spondylodiskitis may be initially dominated by the primary infection. Consequently, a considerable delay between disease onset and diagnosis may develop. Clinicians should suspect spondylodiskitis in patients with new or worsening back or neck pain accompanied by fever, neurologic symptoms, a recent bacteremia, endocarditis, or other infection symptoms. Pain caused by spondylodiskitis may be misdiagnosed as a degenerative process, back strain, osteoporotic fracture, herniated disk, spinal stenosis, inflammatory conditions, or metastatic disease. Initial misdiagnosis is common in elderly patients, especially in the absence of fever. Clinicians should maintain a high index of suspicion in patients with back and neck pain given the nonspecific array of symptoms.

Hematologic and Biochemical Markers

In general, leukocytosis, neutrophilia, and elevated erythrocyte sedimentation rate (ESR) and C-reactive protein (CRP) suggest a pyogenic infection. Although ESR and CRP are sensitive inflammatory markers for infection, and are elevated in the majority of the spondylodiskitis cases, they lack specificity. CRP is a more sensitive parameter than ESR, and it provides a more accurate reflection of the response to the treatment. The leukocyte count is the least useful among the inflammatory markers and is elevated in only one third to one half of the affected patients. Approximately 70% of the spondylodiskitis patients may be anemic, and about half have a raised alkaline phosphatase serum value. Apart from the inflammatory markers, serological tests such as interferon-γ release assay and seroagglutination assay may be performed in suspected tuberculosis and brucellosis infections.

Imaging

The first diagnostic procedure in patients with back or neck pain is often conventional radiography (CR). However, the sensitivity and specificity of radiography for diagnosing spondylodiskitis is low. In the initial phase, there are usually no CR changes. The earliest radiographic signs of spondylodiskitis can develop 2 to 8 weeks after the initial symptoms and may consist of narrowing of the disk space, blurred outlines of the vertebral end plates, loss of end-plate margins, and osteolysis. At later stages, progression of the infection can reveal further destruction of the vertebral body, reactive changes with new bone formation, and sclerosis. Although upright radiographs can be negative in the early phase, the initial CR is useful as a baseline image to detect deformities or ankylosis of the affected levels and to refer to for comparisons during follow-up (**Fig. 6.1**).

Magnetic resonance imaging (MRI) is the diagnostic procedure of choice and is recommended in all patients with suspected spondylodiskitis. MRI has a high sensitivity (96%) and specificity (92%).[5] The MRI protocol can consist of several standard sequences including spin echo (T1- and T2-weighted), gradient echo (T2-weighted), fat signal suppression, short tau inversion recovery (STIR), and contrast-enhanced images. Signs of infection consist of areas of low signal within the vertebral body, loss of end-plate margins, and disruption of cortical continuity on T1-weighted images. The inflammatory tissue generates a strong signal and a hyperintense disk on T2-weighted images in contrast to degenerative changes, where the intervertebral disk is usually hypointense due to dehydration. Fluid-sensitive MRI sequences

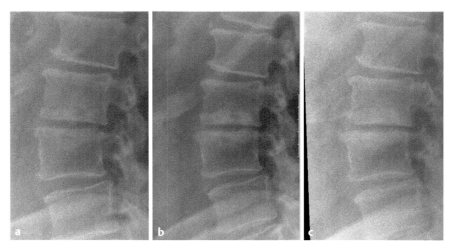

Fig. 6.1 Radiographic follow-up of pyogenic spondylodiskitis L2–L3 in a 67-year-old man. **(a)** X-rays at diagnosis and at **(b)** 3 and **(c)** 6 months. **(a)** Narrowing of disk height and blurring of the end plates at diagnosis. **(b)** Three months after diagnosis, further loss of disk height and sclerosis of the end plates. **(c)** Six months after diagnosis, an increase in sclerosis and the first signs of anterior osseous bridging.

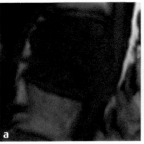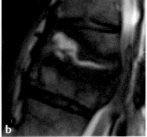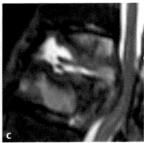

Fig. 6.2 Magnetic resonance imaging (MRI) of T8–T9 pyogenic spondylodiskitis in an 80-year-old woman. **(a)** T1-weighted image: low signal within the vertebral body, loss of end-plate margins, disruption of cortical continuity, and destruction of the vertebral body. **(b)** T2-weighted image: hyperintense signal in the disk and in the adjacent vertebrae. **(c)** Short tau inversion recovery (STIR) T2-weighted image: highly sensitive for detecting early inflammatory changes; signal distribution is similar to that on standard T2-weighted images.

such as STIR and fat-saturated T2-weighted images are highly sensitive for detecting early inflammatory changes.[6] Furthermore, additional pre- and postcontrast fat-suppressed T1-weighted images enable differentiating between vascularized (hyperemic osseous and soft tissue) and nonvascularized, necrotic (abscesses, bone sequesters) inflammatory components. Despite the high sensitivity, MRI findings in early spondylodiskitis may be atypical and overlap with findings in other conditions such as Modic type 1 changes, Schmorl's node, disk extrusion, malignancy, and acute end-plate fractures. Therefore, it remains important to correlate these early MRI findings with clinical history and laboratory tests (**Fig. 6.2**).

When it is not possible to request an MRI because the patient has implantable cardiac devices, cochlear implants, or claustrophobia, fluorine-18 fluorodeoxyglucose positron emission tomography (FDG-PET) can be an excellent alternative diagnostic procedure. Because there is hardly any physiological uptake of FDG in the spinal column, the increased glucose metabolism in activated inflammatory cells are imaged as a "hot spot" in the PET scan. Furthermore, FDG-PET can distinguish between initial spondylodiskitis and common degenerative changes in the adjacent bone. Overall, FDG-PET has a very high sensitivity and specificity in diagnosing spondylodiskitis and also facilitates assessment of abscesses and the extent of the

infection by combining it with computed tomography (CT). However, tumors also have an increased uptake of FDG, and therefore differentiation between malignant processes and spondylodiskitis may be difficult.

When MRI and FDG-PET are unavailable or impossible, other imaging modalities such as CT or gallium-67/technetium-99 bone scans can be requested. Although CT's sensitivity and specificity are inferior to those of MRI in detecting spondylodiskitis, CT can provide details on disease progression, bone destruction, sequestration of the end plate, cortical erosions, and sclerosis. CT imaging of nervous structures and soft tissues may be limited. However, contrast enhancement can provide good imaging of paravertebral abscesses, and CT guidance for percutaneous diagnostic needle biopsy and drainage of abscesses can help identify the causative microorganism. Nuclear medicine techniques such as gallium-67 or technetium-99 bone scan or single photon emission computed tomography (SPECT) also have a high sensitivity in diagnosing spondylodiskitis. The inflammatory changes or increased bone remodeling in spondylodiskitis results in spots with increased radiotracer accumulation in the spine. Due to this high sensitivity, a normal bone scan provides reliable evidence for the absence of inflammation. However, degenerative changes or tumors can produce false-positive results. Consequently, the specificity of these techniques is low, and increased uptake

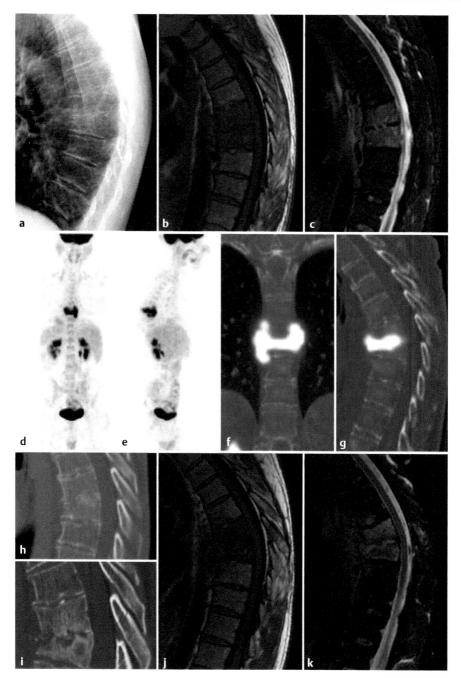

Fig. 6.3 Different imaging techniques of a 53-year-old patient with a pyogenic spondylodiskitis T7–T8 with unknown pathogen. **(a)** Early conventional radiography (CR) shows narrowing of the disk space and blurred outlines of the end plates. An MRI in an early phase showing signal changes within the vertebral body and loss of end-plate margins on **(b)** T1 images with a hyperintense small area of the disk on the **(c)** STIR. Positron emission tomography (PET) **(d,e)** combined with computed tomography (CT) **(f,g)** showing an abnormal hot spot at the T7–T8 disk level indicative of spondylodiskitis. **(h)** CT images at an early phase and during CT-guided biopsy for the second time **(i),** showing initial narrowing of the disk space and subsequent disease progression with bone destruction, cortical erosions, and sclerosis. MRI during disease progression with cortical disruption on **(j)** T1 images and **(k)** a strong signal, with a hyperintense disk area on STIR images.

can be only suggestive for spondylodiskitis. Combining these techniques with CT imaging results in a higher specificity.

In summary, several imaging techniques can be used to diagnose spondylodiskitis, but each of these techniques has limitations. Whereas MRI remains the preferred diagnostic procedure, alternative methods such as FDG-PET, CT, gallium-67 scans, technetium-99 scans, and CR can be used when MRI is not possible or unavailable (**Fig. 6.3**).

Cultures

Identification of the responsible microorganism and determination of its susceptibility for antibiotic treatment are essential. Unless clinical circumstances such as severe sepsis dictate otherwise, empiric antibiotic therapy should not be started before every effort is made to obtain adequate cultures.[3] It is recommended to obtain both aerobic and anaerobic blood cultures.[3] In a systematic review, blood cultures resulted in the isolation of the pathogen in 30 to 78% of the patients.[7] It has been suggested that blood cultures directly following diskovertebral biopsy may result in a higher yield of positive cultures.[8]

Another way to identify the microorganism is to perform CT-guided fine-needle biopsies and percutaneous or open surgical biopsies. When blood cultures are negative and clinical circumstances allow postponing antibiotic treatment, local sampling is recommended.[3] Although CT-guided biopsies are the least invasive and the preferred initial method for local sampling, they provide a relatively low quantity of tissue, which can lead to negative results. So far, isolation of the microorganism from biopsies ranges from 30 to 91% in the literature.[9–12] Therefore, it is recommended that a second biopsy be performed in patients with suspected spondylodiskitis with negative blood cultures and the original image-guided biopsy.[3] These second biopsies should also be tested for more difficult to grow microorganisms. Extended culture times can help to detect low-virulence organisms. Molecular methods such as 16S rRNA polymerase chain reaction (PCR)

and sequencing can also be helpful for diagnosing spondylodiskitis in suspected cases and for determining the pathogen.[13] Percutaneous endoscopic diskectomy or open excisional biopsy can be considered because culture positivity is higher with surgical sampling. The diagnostic yield can be further improved by obtaining more than one specimen for culture and histopathological investigation. If antibiotic treatment was already started and clinical improvement stagnates, discontinuation of the antibiotics for some days is recommended before the biopsies are taken. When antibiotic treatment fails, clinicians should also be aware of a possible superinfection by another microorganism. Therefore, it is recommended to obtain new cultures in case of a relapse of pyogenic spondylodiskitis, including cultures for tuberculosis.

Conservative Treatment

Eradication of infection, pain relief, and restoration and preservation of the structure and function of the spine are the main aims of the treatment of spondylodiskitis.[14] The vast majority of patients with pyogenic spondylodiskitis can be treated conservatively.[2] Conservative treatment consists of antibiotic treatment, analgesia, and limitation of physical activities. Adequate antibiotic treatment based on the susceptibility spectrum of the identified microorganism and appropriate duration of antibiotic treatment is essential for successful conservative management. In general, 6 weeks of antibiotic treatment is considered to be sufficient for pyogenic spondylodiskitis.[3,15] Two weeks of intravenous treatment followed by 4 weeks of oral administration of antibiotics with a high bioavailability in bone is a common treatment strategy. Duration of antibiotic treatment should be adjusted to the identified microorganism and patient characteristics.[16] The best available evidence suggests that 6 weeks of antibiotic treatment is sufficient for the treatment of pyogenic spondylodiskitis caused by *Staphylococcus aureus*,[15,17] whereas more than 8 weeks of antibiotic treatment is suggested for methicillin-resistant *S. aureus* (MRSA).[18] Additionally

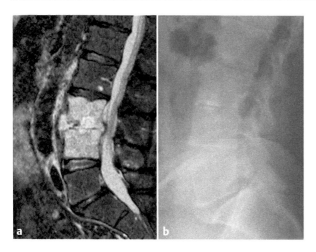

Fig. 6.4 Conservative treatment of pyogenic spondylodiskitis L3–L4 in a 52-year-old patient caused by *Propionibacterium acnes*. The patient was treated with 6 weeks of antibiotic treatment. **(a)** The MRI scan was made at diagnosis. **(b)** CR after 6 weeks of antibiotic treatment showing ongoing fusion at the L3–L4 intervertebral disk.

a reduced relapse rate was reported for daptomycin instead of vancomycin treatment in spondylodiskitis-caused MRSA.[19] Longer antibiotic treatment is suggested for immunocompromised patients, but clinical studies supporting this suggestion are lacking. If the causative microorganism cannot be identified, the patient should be treated empirically based on local epidemiological data regarding the most common pathogens and susceptibility.

Limitation of physical activity is thought to reduce pain and progression of the disease and is therefore often part of the standard treatment of spondylodiskitis.[2] Nevertheless, there is no evidence that bed rest or limitation of physical activity has any effect on the clinical course of the disease. Furthermore, there is no evidence that a brace or orthosis reduces pain or can prevent deformity. Despite the lack of evidence regarding ambulation and the use of an orthosis, a pragmatic approach with bed rest until the inflammation markers start to decrease and ambulation on an as tolerated basis with a brace is a common strategy used by many experts in the field[16] (**Fig. 6.4**).

Surgical Treatment

Although the majority of spondylodiskitis patients can be treated conservatively, there are clear indications for surgical management in some cases. Neurologic deficits due to compression of the spinal cord or the cauda equina, spinal instability or progressive deformity, and failure of conservative management are indications for surgical intervention. The need for an open biopsy can also be considered as a relative indication for surgical management.

The primary aim of surgery is decompression of neural tissue in case of deficit, debridement of the infected intervertebral disk, and stabilization of the affected segment(s). Historically, anterior debridement and stabilization has been the standard surgical treatment for spondylodiskitis, whereas posterior stabilization has been used as an adjunct to this procedure.[14] We strongly advise against decompression without stabilization because this commonly requires additional stabilizing surgery.[16] Nowadays, with the availability of modern spinal surgery techniques, many surgeons prefer a posterior-only approach in which decompression, debridement, and stabilization can be performed adequately in a single surgery. If the destruction of the vertebrae is so extensive that it results in instability or progressive deformity, reconstruction of the vertebral column is indicated. Both polyetheretherketone (PEEK) and titanium cages can safely be used for reconstruction in cases with severe destruction of the vertebrae.[14,16] There is no difference in clinical outcome between open anterior, posterior, or 360-degree techniques as long as the primary aims of the surgery are met.[16] Therefore, determining the approach should be based on the surgical experience of the attending surgeon and on the patient and disease characteristics. If decompression of multiple levels is required, a posterior approach might be more suitable.

More modern surgical strategies, such as percutaneous procedures, hold great promise. Recent studies of posterior percutaneous stabilization with pedicle screws with or without transpedicular drainage show similar results with regard to mortality and relapse rate and a better functional outcome than with an open posterior approach.[16] Moreover, there are even some indications that posterior percutaneous procedures could lead to earlier mobilization, faster recovery, and better quality of life when compared with conservative treatment[20] (**Figs. 6.5, 6.6, 6.7**).

Multidisciplinary Treatment

Diagnosis and management of spondylodiskitis can be complex and should only be done in a medical center that has enough resources to obtain a full workup, where the physicians have the experience to recognize the indications for surgical management, and where there is access to surgical care within an appropriate time frame when needed. Spondylodiskitis should be treated by a multidisciplinary team consisting of consultants from internal medicine, infectious disease, microbiology, and spine surgery. Cases should be discussed by the entire team when the workup is completed and the initial treatment is started. Additionally, the response to the initiated treatment should be evaluated at standard time points (e.g., 2, 6, and 12 weeks, and 1 year). CRP and CR images are the most important investigations to monitor the response to the initiated treatment or to detect relapse of the infection or occurrence of spinal deformities. Follow-up for at least 1 year after diagnosis is advised. Follow-up imaging with MRI should be performed only if indicated. Routine MRI scans can only be confusing and are not advised due to poor correlation between MRI changes and the response to treatment.[3,4]

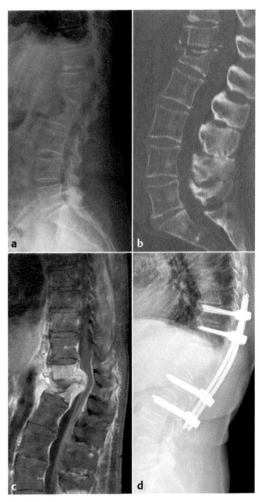

Fig. 6.5 Pyogenic spondylodiskitis T12-L1 in a 69-year-old patient with a partial cauda syndrome caused by Streptococcus pneumoniae. **(a,b)** CR and CT showing destruction and sequestration of the end plates with kyphosis at T12-L1. **(c)** Postcontrast fat-suppressed T1-weighted MRI showing hyperemic bone and soft tissues in the spinal canal with stenosis at the level of the conus medullaris. **(d)** Lateral CR after percutaneous fixation of T10-L3 and an open decompression T12-L1 with fusion of the intervertebral disk T12-L1.

Clinical Outcome

There are few published studies of the long-term outcomes of spondylodiskitis treatment. Overall mortality of ~ 5% is commonly reported, with a range of 1 to 11%. Similar mortality rates are reported for conservatively

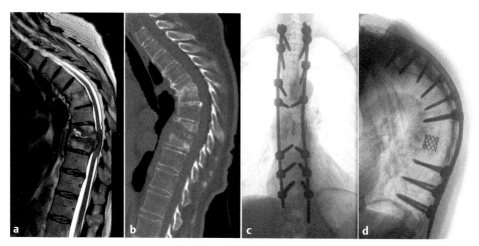

Fig. 6.6 Pyogenic spondylodiskitis at T8-T9 in an 81-year-old patient caused by *Streptococcus pneumoniae*. The patient was known to have had a spondylodiskitis at T5–T6 before this presentation. At presentation, the patient had several months of disabling back pain and progressive neurologic deficits. **(a,b)** MRI and CT at diagnosis show severe destruction of T8–T9 and compression of the spinal cord. The patient was treated with a laminectomy at T8–T9, posterolateral debridement of T8–T9, and insertion of a cage followed by an spondylodesis from T2 to T12. **(c,d)** CR at 1-year follow-up.

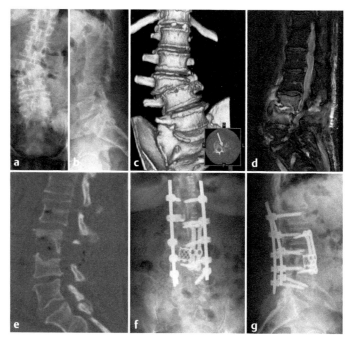

Fig. 6.7 Pyogenic spondylodiskitis L3–L4 caused by *Propionibacterium acnes* after microdiskectomy in a 74-year-old patient. **(a,b)** CR and **(c)** CT reconstruction show retrolisthesis at L3-L4 and scoliotic deformity caused by the spondylodiskitis. **(d)** Fast spin echo inversion recovery MRI scan showing abscess formation at the disk level and destruction of the L3 and L4 end plates. **(e)** Postoperative CT after a posterior reconstruction and spondylodesis with debridement of the disk space showing a large anterior bone defect. Three weeks after the posterior spondylodesis and initiation of antibiotic therapy, a secondary procedure was done and an anterior cage was placed to fill the gap. **(f,g)** The CR shows the direct postoperative result.

treated patients and for surgically treated patients.[21] For conservatively treated patients, relapse rates from 0 to 9% have been reported, and additional surgical treatment is required in 0 to 55% of the patients in different series.[16] These findings are similar to those in patients whose initial treatment was surgical (relapse rate 0–10%), and in this group also additional surgery was needed in 0 to 55%.[16] Relapse predominantly occurs shortly after the initial treatment, and 75% of all relapses occur in the first year after treatment.[21] Not much information has been published about the functional outcomes after spondylodiskitis. Children usually have an excellent prognosis with good functional outcome.[21] In adults the prognosis is less favorable, as up to a third of the patients develop chronic back pain after spondylodiskitis.[21] Additionally, the presence of neurologic deficits is a major factor in the functional outcome after spondylodiskitis.

Diagnosis and Treatment of Failure of Initial Management or Relapse

Treatment failure is defined as persisting clinical symptoms or unchanged elevated CRP after 4 weeks of adequate treatment.[3] Additionally, progression of destruction of the vertebrae, progressive deformity, and development of neurologic deficits are an indication that the current treatment is failing. Relapse is defined as an increase in CRP and in clinical symptoms after successful completion of the initial treatment. Failure of conservative treatment is an indication for surgical debridement and stabilization, and a spine surgeon should be consulted. Failure of surgical management often requires re-debridement and additional stabilization. If the patient is treated surgically, new tissue samples for culture and histological evaluation should be obtained, ideally after an interval without antibiotic treatment. In cases of relapse, new cultures should be obtained, and if previous cultures were negative and the

patient was treated empirically, an open biopsy in combination with surgical debridement and stabilization should be considered.

Chapter Summary

Pyogenic spondylodiskitis is often initially misdiagnosed due to the relatively nonspecific array of symptoms. Consequently, clinicians should maintain a high index of suspicion in patients with back and neck pain and should do additional tests when in doubt. Elevated erythrocyte sedimentation rate (ESR) or C-reactive protein (CRP) with or without leukocytosis or neutrophilia suggests a pyogenic infection. MRI is the preferred diagnostic imaging procedure to diagnose spondylodiskitis. Alternative methods such as FDG-PET, CT, gallium-67 scans, technetium-99 scans, and conventional radiograms can be used when MRI is not possible or unavailable. Identification of the specific microorganism causing the infection is essential. Blood cultures should be taken in all patients. When blood cultures are negative and clinical circumstances allow postponing antibiotic treatment, local biopsies are recommended. Overall, clinicians should be aware of a significant risk of false-negative results for all diagnostic tests for spondylodiskitis.

The majority of patients with spondylodiskitis can be treated conservatively. Conservative treatment consists of proper antibiotic administration for at least 6 weeks and limitation of physical activity. The antibiotics should be adjusted based on the susceptibility of the microorganisms and on patient characteristics. Neurologic deficits, deformity, spinal instability, and failure of conservative treatment are indications for surgical management of spondylodiskitis. A relative indication for an open biopsy in combination with surgical stabilization is treatment failure or relapse after empiric antibiotic treatment in culture-negative spondylodiskitis. Up to a third of the patients develop chronic low back pain after biochemically and radiographic successful treatment of spondylodiskitis.

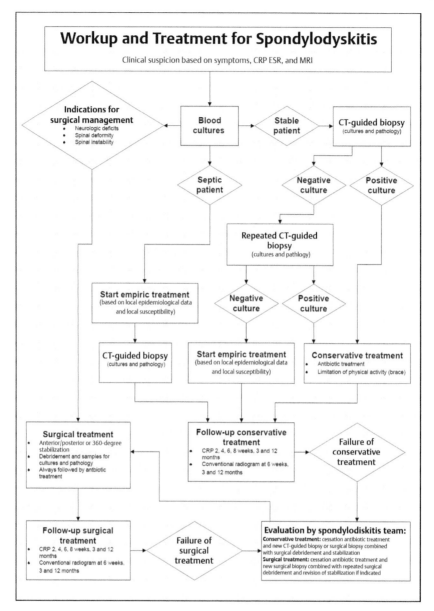

Fig. 6.8 Algorithm for the diagnostic workup and treatment of pyogenic spondylodiskitis. CRP, C-reactive protein; CT, computed tomography; ESR, erythrocyte sedimentation rate; MRI, magnetic resonance imaging.

◆ MRI is the preferred diagnostic imaging test for spondylodiskitis with the highest sensitivity and specificity (**Fig. 6.8**).
◆ Identification of the responsible microorganisms is of prime importance.

◆ At-risk patients might need longer or more aggressive treatment.
◆ Clinicians should know the indications for surgical management.

References

Five Must-Read References

1. Jensen AG, Espersen F, Skinhøj P, Rosdahl VT, Frimodt-Møller N. Increasing frequency of vertebral osteomyelitis following Staphylococcus aureus bacteraemia in Denmark 1980–1990. J Infect 1997;34: 113–118
2. Cheung WY, Luk KD. Pyogenic spondylitis. Int Orthop 2012;36:397–404
3. Berbari EF, Kanj SS, Kowalski TJ, et al. Executive Summary: 2015 Infectious Diseases Society of America (IDSA) Clinical Practice Guidelines for the Diagnosis and Treatment of Native Vertebral Osteomyelitis in Adults. Clin Infect Dis 2015;61:859–863
4. Zimmerli W. Clinical practice. Vertebral osteomyelitis. N Engl J Med 2010;362:1022–1029
5. Modic MT, Feiglin DH, Piraino DW, et al. Vertebral osteomyelitis: assessment using MR. Radiology 1985; 157:157–166
6. Leone A, Dell'Atti C, Magarelli N, et al. Imaging of spondylodiscitis. Eur Rev Med Pharmacol Sci 2012; 16(Suppl 2):8–19
7. Mylona E, Samarkos M, Kakalou E, Fanourgiakis P, Skoutelis A. Pyogenic vertebral osteomyelitis: a systematic review of clinical characteristics. Semin Arthritis Rheum 2009;39:10–17
8. Cherasse A, Martin D, Tavernier C, Maillefert JF. Are blood cultures performed after disco-vertebral biopsy useful in patients with pyogenic infective spondylitis? Rheumatology (Oxford) 2003;42:913
9. Chew FS, Kline MJ. Diagnostic yield of CT-guided percutaneous aspiration procedures in suspected spontaneous infectious diskitis. Radiology 2001;218: 211–214
10. Heyer CM, Brus LJ, Peters SA, Lemburg SP. Efficacy of CT-guided biopsies of the spine in patients with spondylitis—an analysis of 164 procedures. Eur J Radiol 2012;81:e244–e249
11. Michel SC, Pfirrmann CW, Boos N, Hodler J. CT-guided core biopsy of subchondral bone and intervertebral space in suspected spondylodiskitis. AJR Am J Roentgenol 2006;186:977–980
12. Sehn JK, Gilula LA. Percutaneous needle biopsy in diagnosis and identification of causative organisms in cases of suspected vertebral osteomyelitis. Eur J Radiol 2012;81:940–946
13. Sheikh AF, Khosravi AD, Goodarzi H, et al. Pathogen identification in suspected cases of pyogenic spondylodiscitis. Front Cell Infect Microbiol 2017;7:60
14. Guerado E, Cerván AM. Surgical treatment of spondylodiscitis. An update. Int Orthop 2012;36:413–420
15. Bernard L, Dinh A, Ghout I, et al; Duration of Treatment for Spondylodiscitis (DTS) study group. Antibiotic treatment for 6 weeks versus 12 weeks in patients with pyogenic vertebral osteomyelitis: an open-label, non-inferiority, randomised, controlled trial. Lancet 2015;385:875–882
16. Rutges JP, Kempen DH, van Dijk M, Oner FC. Outcome of conservative and surgical treatment of pyogenic spondylodiscitis: a systematic literature review. Eur Spine J 2016;25:983–999
17. Roblot F, Besnier JM, Juhel L, et al. Optimal duration of antibiotic therapy in vertebral osteomyelitis. Semin Arthritis Rheum 2007;36:269–277
18. Park KH, Chong YP, Kim SH, et al. Clinical characteristics and therapeutic outcomes of hematogenous vertebral osteomyelitis caused by methicillin-resistant Staphylococcus aureus. J Infect 2013;67:556–564
19. Rangaraj G, Cleveland KO, Gelfand MS. Comparative analysis of daptomycin and vancomycin in the treatment of vertebral osteomyelitis. Infect Dis Clin Pract 2014;22:219–222
20. Nasto LA, Colangelo D, Mazzotta V, et al. Is posterior percutaneous screw-rod instrumentation a safe and effective alternative approach to TLSO rigid bracing for single-level pyogenic spondylodiscitis? Results of a retrospective cohort analysis. Spine J 2014;14: 1139–1146
21. Gouliouris T, Aliyu SH, Brown NM. Spondylodiscitis: update on diagnosis and management. J Antimicrob Chemother 2010;65(Suppl 3):iii11–iii24

7

Spinal Epidural Abscess

Frank Kandziora, Klaus John Schnake, and Christoph-H. Hoffmann

Introduction

Since its first description in G.B. Morgagni´s landmark work *De sedibus et causis morborum per anatomen indigatis libri quinque*,[1] published in 1761, spinal epidural abscess (SEA) has been a rare entity of infectious disease associated with mortality rates as high as 80 to 100%. High morbidity and mortality rates have been steadily lowered with the advent of surgical decompressive techniques, namely laminectomy, since the early 20th century, and antimicrobial agents since the 1940s, but SEA remains a potentially life-threatening condition; recent publications have cited mortality rates ranging from 2 to 31%.[2,3] Moreover, the incidence of SEA seems to be on the rise: Baker et al[4] reported an annual incidence of 0.2 to 1.2 per 10,000 hospital admissions in 1975, but more recent publications reported remarkably higher rates, reaching 2.5 to 3 per 10,000 hospital admissions.[2] More patients with known risk factors (see below) for the development of SEA are among the reasons for the observed increase in SEA incidence rates.

Etiology

Spinal epidural abscess is an infectious process located in the epidural space of the spine (cervical 15%, thoracic 50%, lumbar 35%[5]), which is initiated by microorganisms that cause an inflammatory response. Typically, *Staphylococcus aureus* is found in specimens from SEA, accounting for 60 to 90% of cases.[6,7] Methicillin-resistant *S. aureus* (MRSA) is also reported with increasing frequency.[7] Other bacterial organisms causing SEA include: *Streptococcus, Escherichia coli, Pseudomonas aeruginosa, Diplococcus pneumoniae, Serratia marcescens,* and *Enterobacter.* In chronic SEA, *Mycobacterium tuberculosis* is found in at least 25% of cases worldwide. Fungal and parasitic infections are seen less frequently. These include *Cryptococcus, Aspergillus, Brucella,* and *Echinococcus.*

There are three patterns of infection of the spinal epidural space:

1. Direct inoculation of microorganisms via spinal procedures (lumbar puncture, dorsal epidural injections, spinal surgery, stab wounds, other types of wounds)
2. Extension of inflammation *per continuitatem* from neighboring infection sites, such as spontaneous spondylodiskitis, psoas abscess, urinary tract infection including pyelonephritis and paranephritic abscess, pharyngeal abscess, mediastinitis, vertebral osteomyelitis, and decubital ulcers
3. Hematogenous spread from other organ systems: among these patterns, skin infections such as furuncles are most common, followed by intravenous (IV) injections (especially with drug abuse), bacterial endo-

carditis, urinary tract infections, respiratory tract infections, and dental and pharyngeal infections

Following the diagnosis of SEA, diagnostic tests to determine the specific site(s) of primary focus of infection are obligatory. Physicians should be aware of the various entry sites and initiate ear, nose and throat (ENT), cardiology, dental, urological, pneumological, abdominal, or dermatological consultations, whenever the cause of infection remains vague.

Patients with one or more of the following conditions are prone to develop SEA due to decreased immunocompetency: diabetes mellitus (15%), chronic renal failure (2%), IV drug abuse (9%), HIV infection (1%), immunosuppressive therapy including long-term corticosteroids (7–16%), and alcoholism (5%). These risk factors are well known,[2,6] and their presence should help to enhance the diagnosis of SEA in patients with precarious symptoms.

Symptomatology

According to Heusner,[8] the initial symptomatology of SEA classically includes back pain, spine tenderness, and fever. In the second stage, spinal irritational signs such as Lasègue's, Kernig's, Lhermitte's, or Brudzinski's signs are encountered, sometimes along with pain radiating into the arms or legs, followed by motor weakness, bowel or bladder dysfunction, and sensory deficits, which can rapidly (< 24 hours) advance into the last stage of paralysis. Unfortunately, the classic triad of early symptoms of SEA is not always present, leaving the physician with a single nonspecific symptom that can be seen in a large number of other spinal and extraspinal conditions. Thus, postoperative SEA may be associated with very few symptoms in the early stages. Additional encephalopathy may draw the attention away from the spine as a source of symptoms.[9] Meticulous attention to the patient's description of symptoms and short-term follow-up combined with diagnostic tests should prevent the physician from making a misdiagnosis or a late diagnosis.

Diagnostic Tests

Laboratory tests, although not specific, can enhance the diagnostic process. Usually, the erythrocyte sedimentation rate is increased by more than 30%, and elevated serum C-reactive protein levels and leukocyte counts are seen especially in patients with acute SEA.

Although elevated leukocyte counts of cerebrospinal fluid (CSF) specimens are often found as a sign of inflammation, we do not encourage the use of lumbar or cervical epidural or CSF puncture close to abscesses as a diagnostic tool for verification of SEA, as these procedures carry a risk of promoting the infection to the intrathecal space.

Radiographic tools are used to confirm the clinical diagnosis. Magnetic resonance imaging (MRI) is the imaging modality of choice. Lesions can be best detected on sagittal and axial images, with a T1-weighted hypointense and T2-weighted hyperintense epidural mass, which typically enhances with gadolinium contrast. Enhancement can include the complete mass, or only patches, or have a ring-like appearance as a result of different stages of the abscess formation.

Other imaging modalities are far less specific: computed tomography (CT) in conjunction with myelography can show epidural mass extensions in patients not amenable for MRI scanning. However, the intrathecal injection of contrast media close to SEA holds a significant risk of distributing the inflammatory process leading to meningitis or myelitis.

Treatment Options

Historically, decompressive laminectomy was the first treatment for SEA. When antibiotics became available in the 1940s, with sulfonamides among the first substances used, nonsurgical therapy became another option in patients without neurocompression.

Nowadays, treatment is unequivocally surgical in most cases of SEA, especially in the presence of a neurologic deficit, followed by antibiotic treatment (initially empirical, secondarily specific to the causative microorganism) as soon as specimens for microbiological examination have been collected.

There is good evidence in the literature that surgery plus antibiotic treatment is superior to antibiotic treatment alone, even if no neurologic deficit is noted upon presentation, and that early surgery is superior to late surgery.[5,10–15]

Patients considered unable to undergo surgical therapy, or those with persisting complete neurologic deficit lasting longer than 48 hours, with little concern about an ascending lesion, or those who are neurologically stable and lack risk factors that portend the failure of medical treatment may be initially treated with antibiotics alone and close clinical monitoring.[5]

Surgical evacuation of pus is generally achieved by laminectomy, which enables a wide posterior decompression of the thecal sac and spinal cord. Posterior decompression is viable for anteriorly, posteriorly, and circumferentially located SEA, because all these locations can be reached without significant distortion of the thecal sac or spinal cord. If an anterior SEA is associated with spondylodiskitis or vertebral osteomyelitis, which by itself is recommended to be treated with anterior or lateral diskectomy or corpectomy together with anterior/lateral instrumentation, anterior decompression may be considered through the opening of the epidural space. However, this procedure carries a risk of disseminating the infectious process to the retropharyngeal, mediastinal, pleural, or retroabdominal space. Surgical principles for treatment of vertebral osteomyelitis and spondylodiskitis should be followed (see Chapter 6).

The exact extent of surgical decompression is tailored to the lesion as depicted by MRI, with multiple levels of involvement requiring longer decompressions. But multilevel decompressions can lead to instability and thus require a simultaneous stabilization of the vertebral column. Attempts to reduce the size of the decompression, and thereby potentially reduce the chances for postoperative instability by choosing minimally invasive techniques, have been reported only in small case series with comparable results of recurrence and residual abscess.[16,17] Laminotomy and laminoplasty have been used, together with open surgical irrigation of the epidural space from one or more entry points, in multilevel SEA. CT- or fluoroscope-guided percutaneous catheter insertion with irrigation has been used predominantly in children, but the case numbers remain small.[5] In light of these studies, percutaneous CT-guided aspiration is discouraged due to the risk of intrathecal dissemination and the possibility of inadequate decompression due to the remaining solid fragments of the abscess formation.

Following laminectomy, the abscess wall is opened using microhooks. Pus or inflammatory tissue available from the lesion is harvested for microbiological cultures. Greater manipulations to resect the abscess wall must be avoided, as this might lead to (new) neurologic deficits. Irrigation with Ringer's solution decreases the concentration of microorganisms and inflammatory substances and should be used extensively. Antibiotic additions (e.g., gentamicin) can be used at the discretion of the surgeon, but no evidence citing any advantages exists. Ultrasound may guide the surgeon to remnants of granulation tissue that may still compress the thecal sac. A subfascial extraspinal suction drain can be inserted for evacuation of pus or blood. Continuous postoperative irrigation and suction should be reserved for recurrent cases, as irrigation may lead to dural compression.

Instrumented stabilization is warranted in all cases, where postoperative instability is deemed possible, especially in cases of simultaneous spondylodiskitis and vertebral osteomyelitis.

Antibiotic therapy is the second mainstay of SEA treatment. Selection of an appropriate agent depends on the microorganism found in the SEA specimen. The yield of the surgical specimen is fairly low (~ 40%), especially in chronic lesions. In these cases, blood cultures taken preoperatively may increase the likelihood of finding the causal microorganism. Because *S. aureus* is the most likely microorganism, third-generation cephalosporins are used as the empirical antibiotic, and vancomycin is used in cases where MRSA is not ruled out. If SEA is combined with spondylodiskitis or vertebral osteomyelitis, bone-penetrating agents should be considered, such as clindamycin. The selection of the appropriate antibiotic agents should also be based on the microorganisms that are typically the underlying cause, whether the cause is diverticulitis or a urinary tract infection. If in doubt, consult a microbiologist.

Antibiotic therapy should be continued for at least 3 to 4 weeks. Bioavailability should be considered in the choice of the antibiotic agent, when switching from IV to peroral administration. Most authors suggest a period of 6 to 8 weeks for treatment. Discontinuation is possible when clinical symptoms and signs have subsided and laboratory findings (erythrocyte sedimentation rate, C-reactive protein) have returned to normal levels. However, follow-up laboratory tests should be performed for a couple of weeks to rule out recurrences. Follow-up MRI is only helpful in patient who do not respond adequately to antibiotic therapy and in whom recurrence is known or suspected, as MRI reliably depicts reduction of the abscess size.[18]

Outcome

The outcome of SEA is mostly determined by its mortality and morbidity in terms of neurologic recovery. There is a paucity of studies examining the resolution of back pain and tenderness or shedding light on recurrence rates.

The introduction of laminectomy and of antimicrobial substances has significantly affected mortality rates. Before 1900, mortality was as high as 80 to 100%. From 1900 to the mid-20th century, mortality was gradually reduced to around 30 to 40%, and since then mortality has been roughly constant at around 0% to 20%.[2,6]

The timing of surgical decompression has an impact on the neurologic outcome. Procedures performed within 24 hours of diagnosis are more likely to turn severe neurologic deficits into slight deficits, and to alleviate slight deficits so that the patient becomes neurologically intact. If surgery was performed late (> 36 hours), outcomes are unequivocally worse, with unchanged neurologic deficits and death occurring more often.[5]

The outcome likely depends on the effectiveness of the antibiotic therapy. In patients with MRSA, outcomes have been reported to be inferior to those in patients without MSSA.

Another factor influencing the outcome is the patient's immunocompetency. There is a correlation between sepsis and death on the one hand, and between sepsis and late surgery on the other. Multiple comorbidities are thought to influence the outcome as well.

Illustrative Case

A 77-year-old woman had multiple spinal fusions for degenerative spondylolisthesis and adjacent segment disease: L5-S1 in 2010, L3-L4 and L4-L5 in 2014, and L2-L3 in 2016. Five weeks after the last operation, she developed low back pain of increasing intensity. Apart from a slight right-sided foot extensor paresis (M4+), which resulted from the first surgery, she did not show any neurologic deficit. Plain x-ray exams of the lumbar spine did not reveal dislocations or loosening of the implants. Leukocyte count was elevated at 11,200 cells/mm^3, and C-reactive protein was elevated at 4.85 mg/dL (reference < 0.3 mg/dL). An MRI scan of the lumbar spine revealed epidural masses dorsal to and compressing the thecal sac reaching from T11 to L2 (**Fig. 7.1**). The patient underwent an urgent decompression (laminectomy T11 to L2 with removal of epidural pus. Additionally, the instrumented stabilization was extended from L2 to T10 with cement augmentation of T10 and T11 pedicle screws.

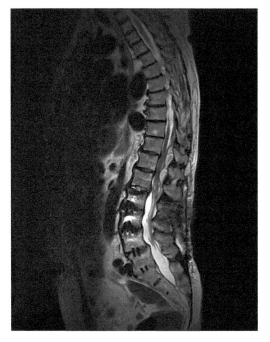

a

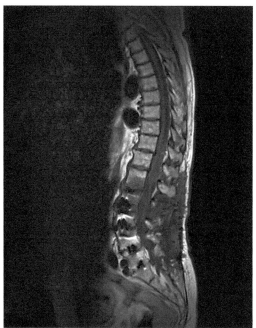

b

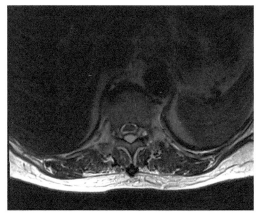

c

Fig. 7.1 (a) Sagittal T2-weighted, **(b)** sagittal T1-weighted, and **(c)** axial T2-weighted lumbar magnetic resonance imaging scans showing dorsal epidural mass located at multiple thoracic and lumbar levels following multilevel spinal stabilization and fusion.

The postoperative lumbar spine plain radiographs (**Fig. 7.2**) depict the extent of the laminectomy. Microbiological cultures from the surgery site grew *Staphylococcus auricularis* and *Staphylococcus hominis*, which are sensitive to ciprofloxacin and clindamycin. These two antibiotics were prescribed for 12 weeks. The patient then made an uneventful recovery and was discharged on the 13th postoperative day with a leukocyte count of $7.700/mm^3$ and C-reactive protein of 4.53 mg/dL. At the follow-up 2 months later, leukocyte counts were normal, as was the C-reactive protein (< 0.3 mg/dL). The patient was free of pain, but the slight paresis remained unchanged.

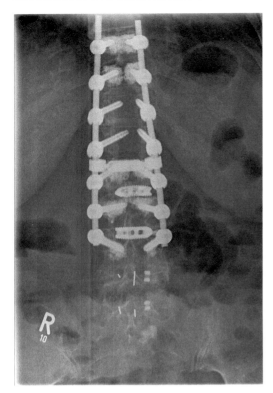

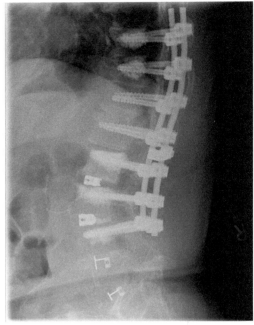

b

Fig. 7.2 Postoperative lumbar x-ray. **(a,b)** The anteroposterior view reveals the extent of the decompressive laminectomy.

a

Pearls

- The classic triad consists of pain, fever, and back tenderness.
- Early surgery with decompression and stabilization in selected cases is the mainstay of therapy.
- Often, extensive irrigation at the abscess site is more effective than complete resection of abscess walls, especially in cases of multisegmental extension of the epidural abscess.

Pitfalls

- Do not overlook multiple lesions; whole spine MRI may be warranted.
- Treatment of the underlying cause is essential; take multiple blood cultures preoperatively, and consult with other subspecialties to locate the possible entry sites.
- Discontinue antibiotic therapy only if complete remission of the inflammatory process is confirmed clinically, radiologically, and by laboratory tests.

References
Five Must-Read References

1. Morgagni GB. De sedibus et causis morborum per anatomen indigatis libri quinque. *Venetiis, Ex Typographia Remondiniana.* Venice, 1761. https://archive.org/details/desedibusetcausi00morg

2. Sendi P, Bregenzer T, Zimmerli W. Spinal epidural abscess in clinical practice. QJM 2008;101:1–12

3. Pereira CE, Lynch JC. Spinal epidural abscess: an analysis of 24 cases. Surg Neurol 2005;63(Suppl 1):S26–S29

4. Baker AS, Ojemann RG, Swartz MN, Richardson EP Jr. Spinal epidural abscess. N Engl J Med 1975;293:463–468

5. Tuchman A, Pham M, Hsieh PC. The indications and timing for operative management of spinal epidural abscess: literature review and treatment algorithm. Neurosurg Focus 2014;37:E8

6. Reihsaus E, Waldbaur H, Seeling W. Spinal epidural abscess: a meta-analysis of 915 patients. Neurosurg Rev 2000;23:175–204, discussion 205

7. Bond A, Manian FA. Spinal epidural abscess: a review with special emphasis on earlier diagnosis. BioMed Res Int 2016;2016:1614328

8. Heusner AP. Nontuberculous spinal epidural infections. N Engl J Med 1948;239:845–854

9. Greenberg MS. Spinal epidural abscess. In: Greenberg MS, ed. Handbook of Neurosurgery, 7th ed. New York: Thieme; 2010:376–380

10. Roßbach BP, Niethammer TR, Paulus AC, et al. Surgical treatment of patients with spondylodiscitis and neurological deficits caused by spinal epidural abscess (SEA) is a predictor of clinical outcome. J Spinal Disord Tech 2014;27:395–400

11. Farber SH, Murphy KR, Suryadevara CM, et al. Comparing outcomes of early, late, and non-surgical management of intraspinal abscess. J Clin Neurosci 2017;36:64–71

12. Suppiah S, Meng Y, Fehlings MG, Massicotte EM, Yee A, Shamji MF. How best to manage the spinal epidural abscess? A current systematic review. World Neurosurg 2016;93:20–28

13. Patel AR, Alton TB, Bransford RJ, Lee MJ, Bellabarba, CB, Chapman JR. Spinal epidural abscesses: risk factors, medical versus surgical treatment, a retrospective review of 128 cases. Spine J 2014;14:326–330

14. Alton TB, Patel AR, Bransford RJ, Bellabarba C, Lee MJ, Chapman JR. Is there a difference in neurologic outcome in medical versus early operative management of cervical epidural abscesses? Spine J 2015;15:10–17

15. Connor DE Jr, Chittiboina P, Caldito G, Nanda A. Comparison of operative and nonoperative management of spinal epidural abscess: a retrospective review of clinical and laboratory predictors of neurological outcome. J Neurosurg Spine 2013;19:119–127

16. Parkinson JF, Sekhon LH. Surgical management of spinal epidural abscess: selection of approach based on MRI appearance. J Clin Neurosci 2004;11:130–133

17. Löhr M, Reithmeier T, Ernestus RI, Ebel H, Klug N. Spinal epidural abscess: prognostic factors and comparison of different surgical treatment strategies. Acta Neurochir (Wien) 2005;147:159–166, discussion 166

18. Veillard E, Guggenbuhl P, Morcet N, et al. Prompt regression of paravertebral and epidural abscesses in patients with pyogenic discitis. Sixteen cases evaluated using magnetic resonance imaging. Joint Bone Spine 2000;67:219–227

8

Spinal Tuberculosis: Pathogenesis, Clinical Features, and Investigations

Rishi M. Kanna, Ajoy Prasad Shetty, and S. Rajasekaran

Introduction

Chronic infections of the vertebral column are usually granulomatous and are caused by mycobacteria, fungi, and *Brucella* species. Among these, tuberculous infection of the spine is the most common. Due to the high vascularity of the vertebral marrow, the tuberculous bacilli have a predilection to afflict the vertebral column, which is the second most common site of tubercular infection after the lungs. Tuberculous infection of the spine usually happens secondary to a primary infection elsewhere, such as the lungs, lymph nodes, kidneys, or the gastrointestinal tract.

Typical symptoms of spinal tuberculosis (TB) include chronic pain at the affected site associated with constitutional symptoms of fever, malaise, and weight loss. In advanced stages of the disease, kyphotic deformity and neurologic deficit can develop. Diagnosis is usually straightforward in endemic regions based on the typical symptoms and signs. But confirmation of the diagnosis through appropriate investigations is essential in view of the growing incidence of drug-resistant TB. There is also a possibility of other pathologies such as pyogenic infections, fungal spondylitis, lymphoproliferative disorders, and spinal metastasis, which may have a similar presentation. A combination of diagnostic tests, including radiographs, magnetic resonance imaging (MRI), the GeneXpert test, tuberculous culture, and histopathological examination, is helpful in confirming the diagnosis. Antitubercular chemotherapy is the mainstay of treatment that has significantly improved the outcome for patients. Although most patients are treated only with chemotherapy, surgery is indicated in specific situations, such as extensive destruction, spinal instability, and gross neurologic deficit. Currently, co-infections with human immunodeficiency virus (HIV) and the drug-resistant TB are major stumbling blocks in the global war against TB.

Epidemiology

Despite significant efforts by global health care organizations and governmental disease control programs, the global burden of TB still remains enormous. According to the World Health Organization (WHO) Global TB report in 2015, there were an estimated 10.4 million new (incident) TB cases worldwide.[1] People living with HIV accounted for 1.2 million (11%) of all new TB cases. Six countries accounted for 60% of the new cases: India, Indonesia, China, Nigeria, Pakistan, and South Africa. In 2015, there were an estimated 490,000 new cases of drug-resistant TB, of which India, China, and the Russian Federation accounted for 45% of cases. There were an estimated 1.4 million TB deaths in 2015, and although the number of TB deaths fell by 22% between 2000 and 2015, TB remains one of the top 10 causes of death worldwide in 2015.

India, China, and South Africa share the major burden of spinal TB, too. In the developing parts of the world, the incidence is higher because of the crowded conditions, poor sanitation, reduced access to health care, and the lack of knowledge about TB among the people and the health care workers. In India, there are 6 million radiologically proven cases of TB, of which nearly 0.5 to 1% are vertebral TB.[2] In developed nations, spinal TB seems predominantly distributed among migrants. An epidemiological study of bone and joint TB conducted by Talbot et al[3] in the United Kingdom found that 74% of 756 patients diagnosed with TB were immigrants from the Indian subcontinent.

Pathogenesis

Tuberculosis is caused by a bacillus of the *Mycobacterium tuberculosis* complex, which includes *M. tuberculosis* (the most common), *M. avis, M. bovis,* and *M. intracellulare.* Most infections are caused by the *M. tuberculosis,* which is a slow-growing aerobic bacillus with a lipid and peptidoglycan-rich cell wall, which prevents it from being destroyed by the host immune system.

Vertebral infection usually occurs following hematogenous dissemination of the bacillus from a primary infective focus such as the lungs. Rarely, the bacilli may also travel from the lung to the spine through the paravertebral venous plexus or by lymphatic drainage from the adjoining nodes. Within the spinal column, most infections occur around the lower thoracic and thoracolumbar junction (50–70%), followed by the thoracic spine (20–30%).[4]

Once they reach the vertebral marrow, the bacilli get lodged in the subchondral zone on either side of the disk, because the paradiskal arteries split on either side of the disk to reach the upper and lower end plates of each disk.

This is the "paradiskal" type of infection, and it is the most common pattern of tubercular spinal infection. The intervertebral disk is not involved primarily, but progressive destruction of the vertebral end plates results in direct spread of infection into the disk. Progressive destruction results in collapse of the vertebral body, leading to kyphosis and pathological fractures. Vertebral body collapse can sometimes affect even two or three contiguous vertebral bodies, resulting in severe kyphosis. The combination of kyphosis, pathological collapse with retropulsed bony fragments, and exuberant abscess formation can compress the spinal cord, resulting in a neurologic deficit. Due to the chronic inflammatory response, extensive abscess formation is typical of TB. The abscess contents slowly spread into the epidural, prevertebral, and paravertebral regions and produce characteristic signs and symptoms.

The second most common pattern is called the centrum type, wherein the infection occurs predominantly within one vertebral body, resulting in complete collapse of the body with sparing of the disks on either side. Extensive involvement with complete destruction of many adjacent vertebral bodies is more commonly seen in children, due to the cartilaginous nature of their bones. In severe cases, this presentation may mimic vertebra plana (complete collapse of one vertebral body), which can occur in other conditions such as histiocytosis and spinal tumors. The presence of extensive abscess formation near the collapsed vertebral body and multifocal involvement helps in differentiating this type from other causes of vertebra plana (**Fig. 8.1**).

A third pattern is infection of the posterior elements, wherein the pedicles, facet joints, spinous process, and lamina are affected alone, with sparing of the vertebral body (**Fig. 8.2**). It is uncommon (< 1%). Diagnosis of posterior-element TB is difficult with conventional radiographs alone, and often requires an MRI instead.[5] A fourth pattern, *non-osseous*, is also very rare, characterized by extensive abscess formation without much bony vertebral damage. It is typically described around the sacroiliac joints and the lower lumbar region.

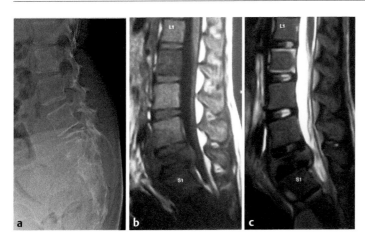

Fig. 8.1 Vertebra plana of the L5 vertebra in a 14-year-old girl. **(a)** Lateral radiograph. Sagittal T1 **(b)** and T2 **(c)** magnetic resonance imaging (MRI) scans show multifocal tuberculosis of L2, L5, and the sacral vertebra.

Microscopic Features

Microscopically, the characteristic pathological lesion of TB is called the tubercle, based on which a confirmatory diagnosis is made by histopathological examination. The tubercle is composed of inflammatory cells, cellular debris, necrotic material, and fibrous tissue. As the bacilli infiltrate the vertebral marrow, the initial immune response is characterized by acute inflammation with polymorphonuclear cells. As the neutrophils are unable to control the tubercular bacilli, a chronic inflammation results, characterized by the infiltration of macrophages and monocytes. Although the tubercle bacilli are phagocytosed by the macrophages, the thick cell wall prevents the death of the bacilli. The macrophages slowly transform into epithelioid cells, which are seen in histopathological images as elongated cells with fine granular, pale eosinophilic cytoplasm and a central, ovoid nucleus. In late stages, the epithelioid cells often merge, forming multinucleated giant cells. These giant cells, referred to as the Langhans giant cells, are one of the characteristic microscopic features of tuberculous lesion. This lesion of TB formed by macrophages, epithelioid cells, Langhans giant cells, and lymphocytes is called the tubercle (from

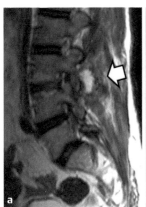
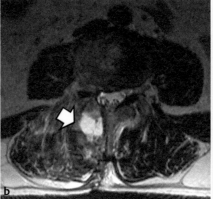
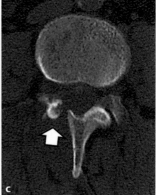

Fig. 8.2 (a) Sagittal T2 MRI of the lumbosacral spine and **(b)** axial T2 sections at the L3–L4 disk show an abscess collection in the right L3–L4 facet joint *(arrow)*. **(c)** Axial computed tomography (CT) image shows destruction of the facet joint and part of the adjoining lamina *(arrow)*.

which the disease gets its name). With progressive destruction, caseation necrosis occurs in the center of the tubercle due to proteolytic destruction by the enzymes released by the macrophages. Adjacent tubercles coalesce to form large abscesses lined by a thin reactive capsule.

Clinical Features

Unlike pyogenic infections of the spine, a tuberculous lesion has a much more insidious onset, and the clinical symptoms often develop over a period of 1 to 2 months. It is a systemic disease, and often infection of multiple organs can coexist. An active concomitant primary tubercular infection in the lungs, lymph nodes, intestines, and kidneys can be present, and should be evaluated through history and clinical examination. Similarly, the lesion can be present in other skeletal regions and in multiple regions of the spine.

Constitutional symptoms of malaise, loss of appetite and weight, evening rise of temperature, and night sweats are typical systemic features of TB. However, in patients with spinal TB, systemic symptoms may not be common. One study reported weight loss in 58% patients, and other constitutional symptoms such as malaise and loss of appetite were observed in 70% of cases.[6]

At the vertebral site of tuberculous infection, the classical clinical presentation involves a tetrad: pain at the affected site, neurologic deficit, abscess formation, and kyphotic deformity.

Pain in Spinal Tuberculosis

Axial pain associated with spinal stiffness is the most common presenting symptom. In different studies, 90 to 100% of patients with spinal TB had back pain.[7] Axial pain in spinal TB is caused by the tubercular inflammatory response, spinal instability (due to destruction of the stabilizing vertebral structures), and periosteal distension (caused by the tubercular abscess). In the early stages, the pain is dull and aching, insidious in onset, and often well controlled by analgesics. However, as spinal instability develops, the intensity of the pain increases. Patients with spinal instability due to thoracic and lumbar TB may need to support their trunk by placing their hands on the couch while sitting ("tripod sign"). Patients with cervical instability due to TB may need to hold their neck with their hands. Due to inflammation and venous engorgement in supine posture, patients with spinal TB have severe pain at night and, in the worst situations, this can manifest as "night cries." The lack of a protective muscle spasm during sleep can result in sudden pathological movement across the destroyed bones, causing severe pain. Radicular pain is an uncommon feature and indicates compression on the nerve roots due to abscess or free bone fragments.

Kyphosis

As the disease progresses, gradual destruction of the vertebral body occurs, which results in a localized kyphotic deformity. The severity of kyphosis varies, depending on the extent of the vertebral body damage. Single (isolated) vertebral collapse results in a knuckle deformity, whereas destruction of several vertebrae results in "gibbus" (collapse of two to three vertebrae) or angular kyphosis (multiple vertebral collapse). The vertebral bodies at the apex of kyphosis can retropulse into the canal, causing neurologic deficit. With progressive destruction and further destabilization, chronic vertebral subluxation and translations can occur, further compromising the spinal canal. Lesions of the cervical and lumbar region tolerate vertebral destruction without much local kyphosis due to their inherent lordosis, whereas thoracic lesions present earlier with significant deformity.

The development and progression of kyphosis differ in children and adults.[8] In adults, the kyphosis progresses only during the active phases of the disease, and the severity of the kyphosis depends mainly on the extent of vertebral body damage. But in children, the kyphosis progresses more rapidly during the active phase because of their soft bones. Further, the kyphosis present at the end of vertebral healing can worsen during the remaining period of growth even after curing the disease. This has been observed in 40% of children in a longitudinal study.[9] Hence, children with healed TB need periodic follow-up until their growth is completed. Rajasekaran[9] has described four spine at-risk signs as indicators for progressive kyphosis; children with two of the signs were found to be at serious risk of a gross increase in deformity.

Cold Abscess

A cold abscess is a diagnostic feature of spinal TB that is present in at least 50% of cases of spinal TB. The cold abscess is a collection of caseous material and inflammatory exudate. Being a chronic infection, there are no characteristic signs of active inflammation such as warmth, and hence the abscess is labeled as "cold." The abscesses initially form within the infective focus and slowly become squeezed along various natural fascial and neurovascular planes. The cold abscess can present clinically at a site remote from the vertebral lesion. It can track along the muscle planes and the perineural, perivascular, subpleural, subperitoneal, and natural areolar tissue spaces. For example, a paravertebral abscess from the thoracolumbar or lumbar vertebral infection tracks along the psoas muscle sheath and can be present bilaterally in various sizes (**Fig. 8.3**). It can track distally through the psoas tendon into the inguinal region or rarely into the thigh or calf region. Abscesses per se are asymptomatic despite some being of enormous size. A superficial abscess can drain through the skin and can be unsightly, whereas deeper abscesses can rarely cause pressure symptoms.

Neurologic Deficit

Neurologic deficit is a serious complication of spinal TB that affects 32 to 76% of patients with spinal TB.[10] An interesting aspect of neurologic involvement in spinal TB is that it can

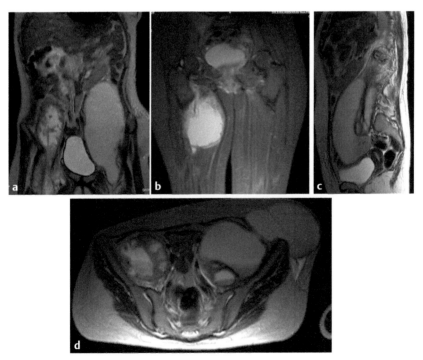

Fig. 8.3 Extensive psoas abscess formation in a patient with lumbar tubercular spondylodiscitis. Coronal T2 MRI demonstrates a huge loculated abscess in the **(a)** iliofemoral region and **(b)** right psoas insertion and medial thigh. **(c)** Sagittal MRI reveals a huge abscess arising from the L2 vertebra and draining into the iliacus muscle. **(d)** Axial T2 MRI of pelvis shows a multiloculated abscess in the right iliac fossa and left iliacus draining into the superficial femoral triangle.

occur both in the active phases of the disease and in the healed stages. In active lesions, it occurs from direct spinal cord compression by tuberculous epidural abscess, granulation tissue, pathological fractures/subluxation, and retropulsion of destroyed bone fragments or sequestrum.

Neurologic deficit can also occur even after complete healing of the disease, especially in children who develop progressive kyphotic deformity in the healed phase. The spinal cord is gradually stretched along the posterior vertebral wall over a bony ridge at the apex of the deformity, resulting in spastic paraparesis. Management of neurologic deficit in the acute and active phases of the disease is less complex and has a good prognosis, whereas late-onset neurologic deficits have a poor prognosis even with surgical treatment.

Cervical spine infection presents with quadriparesis, while thoracic and thoracolumbar lesions manifest as paraparesis. Due to the capacious spinal canal, neurologic deficit is rare in lumbar infection. The earliest neurological manifestation in cord level lesions is a gradual increase in spasticity, which may not be appreciated by the patient. On clinical examination, the patient is typically observed to demonstrate clumsiness and ataxia while walking. As spinal cord compression increases, varying degrees of motor loss and reduction of sensations ensue, and the patient eventually becomes bed bound.

With severe cord compression, there is loss of fine sensation, proprioception, and sphincter control, resulting in flaccid paralysis.

Atypical Spinal Tuberculosis

A patient with TB of the spine who does not present with such typical clinical features as axial pain, constitutional symptoms, kyphosis, neurologic deficit, or typical radiological features is considered to have an atypical presentation. Atypical clinical presentations include symptoms mimicking a prolapsed intervertebral disk, cold abscess without obvious bony lesion, and intraspinal tubercular granulomas manifesting with symptoms of myelopathy. Atypical radiographic presentations include ivory vertebra, circumferential vertebral involvement, and contiguous and noncontiguous multiple vertebral lesions. The incidence and diagnosis of multifocal noncontiguous spinal TB has increased with the availability of whole spine MRI.[11] Although the presenting symptoms and signs are usually due to one particular lesion, multiple noncontiguous lesions can be identified in many patients by MRI of the whole spine. Patients with a systemic infection often have coexistent lesions of the lungs, lymph nodes, and, sometimes, the brain (**Fig. 8.4**).

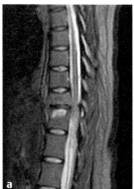
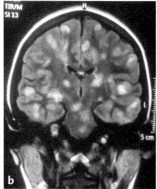
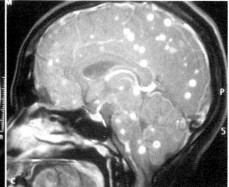

Fig. 8.4 This 22-year-old woman presents with axial mid-back pain and headache. (a) Sagittal T2 MRI shows a tubercular lesion at T11 vertebra. In the same patient, Coronal (b) and sagittal (c) T2 brain images reveal multiple concentric hyperintense regions suggestive of multiple tuberculomas.

Investigations

The diagnosis of spinal TB in endemic regions such as Asia and Africa is usually made based on the typical clinical features and radiological findings. However, with the rising incidence of TB in the West and atypical presentations, the need for confirmatory laboratory serological and microbiological tests is being increasingly recognized. The sensitivity and specificity of the tests vary, and the gold standard confirmation of tubercular infection is through tubercular culture and histopathological examination.

Laboratory Investigations

Tuberculosis being an infectious disease, the standard initial blood tests performed include the blood cell counts, erythrocyte sedimentation rate (ESR), and C-reactive protein (CRP). The total blood counts are expected to be high, with a differential rise in the lymphocyte count (> 30%), but they can be normal. The ESR is a nonspecific investigation for infective conditions and is elevated, generally above 20 mm/h, in 60 to 83% of cases with TB.[12] Serial ESR measurements are helpful in assessing the response to treatment, as persistently elevated values may indicate drug noncompliance, treatment failure, or alternative diagnosis. C-reactive protein is an acute-phase protein and has been found to be elevated in up to 70% of patients with spinal TB. Guo et al[13] studied 67 patients with active spinal TB; the average preoperative ESR was 79.4 ± 35.6 mm/h and the average CRP was 44.3 ± 17.5 mg/L. Both the values showed significant reduction after 8 weeks of antitubercular chemotherapy.

Immune Response Assessment Tests

The Mantoux test, interferon release assay, and immunoglobulin tests are based on the host immune response to TB. The tuberculin skin test (Mantoux) is based on a person's ability to mount a lymphocyte-based immune response (type 4 immunity) to a low-dose tubercular bacillus antigen. A positive test indicates that the person's body has been exposed to the tubercular antigen but it may not confirm an active infection. A negative test would mean that the person's body did not react to the antigen and that latent TB infection is unlikely. In endemic regions, due to the high prevalence of spinal TB, the test can be positive even in patients without active TB.

The interferon-gamma release assay (IGRA) tests are similar to tuberculin skin tests and rely on the principle of detecting a positive immune response in a person exposed to tuberculous bacilli. These are enzyme-linked immunosorbent assay (ELISA) tests measuring the amount of interferon-γ produced in response to *M. tuberculosis* antigens; examples include the QuantiFERON TB and the QuantiFERON TB Gold In-Tube tests. The sensitivity and specificity of these assays vary from 85 to 95%.[14] Similarly, ELISA tests to assess the immunoglobulin M (IgM) and immunoglobulin G (IgG) antibody response to various TB antigens have been described but are no longer recommended for the diagnosis of active TB. Baseline liver function tests are performed before initiating chemotherapy because most antitubercular drugs are potentially hepatotoxic.

Tissue Studies

Analysis of tissue samples obtained from infected foci is a key step in the confirmation of spinal TB. Tissue analysis includes polymerase chain reaction (PCR) analysis, bacterial culture, and histopathological examination.

Polymerase Chain Reaction

Polymerase chain reaction analysis from tissue samples is considered very sensitive and specific for the diagnosis of spinal TB. The Xpert MTB/RIF (*M. tuberculosis*/rifampin) assay is a PCR-based test in which DNA sequences specific for *M. tuberculosis* can be detected in 90 minutes. The test is rapid and also detects genetic mutations associated with rifampin resistance. Studies have shown that this test is highly accurate, and, when compared with culture, it has 88% sensitivity and 98% specificity.[15] It is also the only WHO-recommended rapid diagnostic test for the detection of TB and rifampin resistance. Sharma et al[16] studied 217 patients with suspected spinal TB; the diagnosis was confirmed on the basis of a culture in 145 of the patients (66.8%). Among the cases in which GeneXpert was used, the sensitivity for the detection of *M. tuberculosis* was 93.5% (43/46). Similarly, Held et al[17] performed a prospective clinical study of 69 consecutive adults with suspected spinal TB, wherein the diagnostic accuracy of GeneXpert was compared with a reference standard of liquid culture. The GeneXpert test showed a sensitivity of 95.6% and specificity of 96.2% for spinal TB, and all cases of multidrug-resistant TB (5.8% incidence) were diagnosed accurately with the GeneXpert test.

Bacterial Culture

A positive mycobacterial culture of the infected tissue is the gold standard confirmatory test for TB. It not only confirms the diagnosis, but

also helps to acquire antibiotic sensitivities to guide therapy. Tuberculous lesions in the lungs are multibacillary, whereas in those in osseous tissues, such as the spine, the lesions multiply slowly and contain much fewer organisms (paucibacillary; < 10^4 colony forming units per milliliter). Hence, acid-fast staining of the smear of infected tissue is unlikely to show any bacillus. Thus, it is essential to culture the infected material from infected bone to isolate the organism. Culture results are obtained at 4 to 6 weeks based on which further drug sensitivity testing is performed, especially in patients with drug-resistant TB (**Fig. 8.5**).

Histopathology Examination

The histopathological examination of infected tissue is also useful to make a diagnosis of TB. The typical histopathological findings are large caseating necrotizing granulomatous lesions

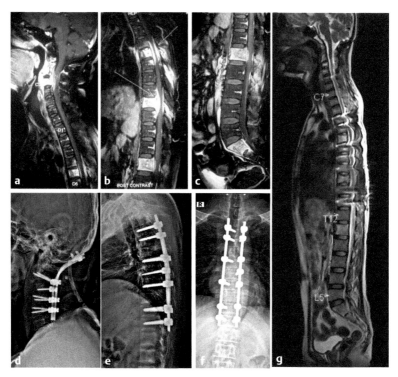

Fig. 8.5 Multidrug resistant, multifocal tuberculosis in a 37-year-old man. (**a–c**) Sagittal cervical, thoracic, and lumbar postcontrast MRI scans reveal multifocal lesions involving the C1-C2, T5, T12, and sacral spine. (**d–f**) Patient underwent debridement, biopsy, and stabilization. Biopsy revealed drug-resistant tuberculosis and hence was treated with second-line drugs for 2 years. (**g**) Follow-up T2 sagittal MRI shows good healing of the lesion.

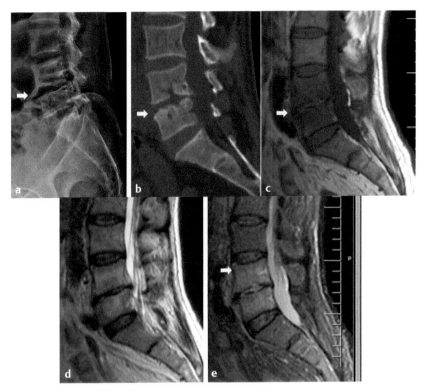

Fig. 8.6 A 42-year-old man presents with axial back pain that was sometimes worse at night. Generally, radiographs show destructive changes only after 3 to 4 weeks of infection. **(a)** Lateral radiograph. Except for mild haziness *(arrow)*, the radiograph is unremarkable. **(b)** Sagittal CT section shows subchondral erosions and areas of lucency *(arrow)*. **(c)** Sagittal T1 hypointensity, **(d)** T2 hyperintensity, and bright signal changes in **(e)** short tau inversion recovery (STIR) sequences indicate diskitis with vertebral marrow edema *(arrow)*.

with epitheloid and multinucleated giant cells with lymphocytic infiltration. The method most widely used to acquire the tissue sample is computed tomography (CT) or fluoroscopy-guided needle/trocar biopsy.

Imaging Studies

Radiographs of the affected area in two planes (anteroposterior [AP] and lateral) are performed as the first line of investigation. The radiographs usually do not show any destruction in the early stages of infection (~ 3–4 weeks) (**Fig. 8.6**). The earliest features observed on plain radiographs are narrowing of the joint space, subchondral lucencies, an indistinct paradiskal margin of vertebral bodies, and vertebral osteoporosis. Further untreated destruction results in vertebral collapse, pathological fractures, local kyphosis, and retropulsion.

Apart from bony destruction, soft tissue shadow of abscesses can be observed in radiographs. In the cervical spine, the normal prevertebral soft tissue shadow in the lateral radiographic view appears widened due to distention of the abscess in the retropharyngeal region. In the thoracic spine, the cold abscess is visible on AP plain radiographs as a fusiform or globular radiodense shadow (bird's nest appearance). Radiographs are good indicators of successful disease healing. Spinal TB heals by bony fusion, and successful healing of disease can be identified in radiographs by the presence of complete bony fusion across the vertebra.

Computed tomography (CT) and magnetic resonance imaging (MRI) can detect lesions at

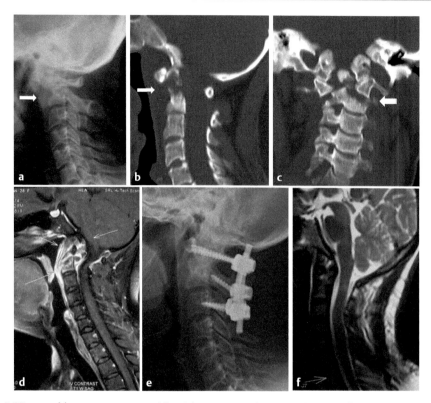

Fig. 8.7 A 28-year-old woman presents with axial neck pain and restricted neck movements. A CT scan is useful in evaluating junctional lesions. **(a)** Lateral radiograph and **(b)** sagittal CT shows destruction of the C1–C2 joint with subluxation *(arrow)*. **(c)** Lateral translation is observed in the coronal CT scan *(arrow)*. **(d)** Sagittal T1 MRI shows an epidural and paravertebral abscess at the cervicothoracic junction. **(e)** The patient was treated with debridement and C1-C3 fusion and chemotherapy. **(f)** Follow-up MRI reveals complete healing of the lesion at 1 year.

an earlier stage. CT is particularly useful in assessing accurately the extent of bony destruction, the levels of surgical fixation, early identification of posterior element involvement, and the identification of TB in certain regions such as the craniovertebral (**Fig. 8.7**), cervicothoracic junction, the sacroiliac joints, and the sacrum, which are not easily defined in the radiographs.

An MRI is the gold standard investigation for evaluating patients with spinal TB. It shows the presence of edema, abscess formation, and granulation tissue within and outside the vertebra. It is useful in demonstrating the extension of disease into soft tissues and the spread of tuberculous abscess in the paravertebral and epidural region. It is the most effective method for demonstrating neural compression and edema within the spinal cord. MRI findings can be useful in differentiating tuberculous spondylitis from pyogenic infections. In a study by Jung et al,[18] the following features favored a diagnosis of tuberculous spondylitis: a well-defined paraspinal abnormal signal, a thin and smooth abscess wall, or a combination of both findings (90% specific); paraspinal or intraosseous abscess; subligamentous spread; involvement of multiple vertebral bodies; and thoracic spine involvement. In patients who presented with a neurologic deficit in the healed stages, the spinal cord showed atrophy with increased signal intensity changes.

The MRI features of spinal TB also provide prognostic information about neurologic recovery. Jain et al[19] observed that patients with relatively preserved cord size with evidence of only myelitis/edema and predominantly fluid collection in the extradural space responded

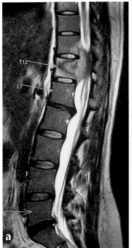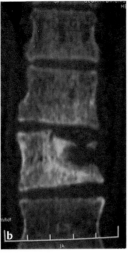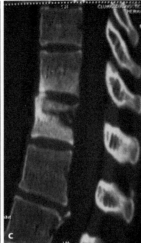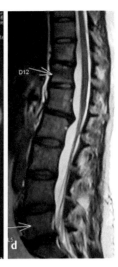

Fig. 8.8 A 38-year-old patient presents with T12 tuberculous spondylitis. **(a–c)** Sagittal and CT images. The patient was treated with a full course of antituberculous chemotherapy and bracing. Follow-up MRI helps in assessing the treatment response in tuberculous spondylodiscitis. **(d)** Sagittal MRI performed at the end of 9 months shows complete disease healing.

well to chemotherapy alone. Patients having significant cord compression and myelomalacia did not show favorable response even after surgical decompression.

The MRI can also be used to assess the response to treatment and regression of the disease (**Fig. 8.8**). The healing of the vertebral lesion is diagnosed on follow-up MRI as complete resolution of marrow edema, replacement of red marrow by fatty infiltration seen as a bright signal on T1- and T2-weighted images, and complete resolution of paravertebral collections.

Chapter Summary

Spinal TB is still prevalent in developing countries. Infection usually develops from hematogenous spread of the organism from a distant primary focus, and uncommonly by direct contiguous spread from adjacent infected organs such as the lungs, kidney, and lymphatics. The focus of infection in the spine starts around the paradiskal regions and can smolderingly extend to multiple adjacent vertebral bodies. The classical clinical features include axial pain at the infected vertebral region, neurologic deficit, varying degrees of kyphosis, and cold abscess. The gold standard investigation to confirm the infection consists of tubercular culture and histopathological examination. However, being a paucibacillary infection, positive detection of bacteria in infected tissues is low; hence, corroborative information from radiographs, MRI, CT, and DNA PCR tests play an important role in making the diagnosis.

Pearls

- The presentation of spinal tuberculous is chronic and innocuous, with chronic axial pain as the main presenting symptom; hence, a high index of clinical suspicion is required for early diagnosis. In suspicious cases, a low threshold for MRI would help in early identification of vertebral infection.
- Multilevel noncontiguous infections are common in the spine; hence, a whole spine MRI is advised in all patients presenting with regional TB.
- Although MRI findings are classic in patients with tuberculous spondylitis, especially in endemic areas, biopsy of the affected bone is essential and has multifold benefits. DNA PCR evaluation, histopathological examination, and tuberculous culture should also be performed.
- The gold standard test results that confirm the diagnosis of spinal TB are a positive tubercular culture and histopathological evidence of tubercular granulomas in infected tissue.

♦ Children with spinal TB can develop late-onset kyphosis despite complete healing of the disease; therefore, periodic follow-up until the completion of growth is required.

♦ Adequate antitubercular chemotherapy ensures good healing in early stage infections without kyphosis and neurologic deficit. As it usually takes 3 to 4 weeks for radiographic changes to be evident, MRI should be performed to diagnose early tuberculous spondylodiskitis.

♦ Immune response tests (Mantoux test, interferon gold assay, IgM and IgG antibody tests) are not helpful in the diagnosis of spinal TB. Positive tests do not indicate the presence of active tubercular infection.

References

Five Must-Read References

1. World Health Organization. Global Tuberculosis Report. Geneva: WHO; 2015
2. Garg RK, Somvanshi DS. Spinal tuberculosis: a review. J Spinal Cord Med 2011;34:440–454
3. Talbot JC, Bismil Q, Saralaya D, Newton DA, Frizzel RM, Shaw DL. Musculoskeletal tuberculosis in Bradford—a 6-year review. Ann R Coll Surg Engl 2007;89:405–409
4. Bajwa GR. Evaluation of the role of MRI in spinal tuberculosis: a study of 60 cases. Pak J Med Sci 2009; 25:944–947
5. Pande KC, Babhulkar SS. Atypical spinal tuberculosis. Clin Orthop Relat Res 2002;398:67–74
6. Hayes AJ, Choksey M, Barnes N, Sparrow OC. Spinal tuberculosis in developed countries: difficulties in diagnosis. J R Coll Surg Edinb 1996;41:192–196
7. Pertuiset E, Beaudreuil J, Lioté F, et al. Spinal tuberculosis in adults. A study of 103 cases in a developed country, 1980–1994. Medicine (Baltimore) 1999;78: 309–320
8. Rajasekaran S. Natural history of Pott's kyphosis. Eur Spine J 2013;22(Suppl 4):634–640
9. Rajasekaran S. The problem of deformity in spinal tuberculosis. Clin Orthop Relat Res 2002;398:85–92
10. Jain AK, Kumar J. Tuberculosis of spine: neurological deficit. Eur Spine J 2013;22(Suppl 4):624–633
11. Kaila R, Malhi AM, Mahmood B, Saifuddin A. The incidence of multiple level noncontiguous vertebral tuberculosis detected using whole spine MRI. J Spinal Disord Tech 2007;20:78–81
12. Hosalkar HS, Agrawal N, Reddy S, Sehgal K, Fox EJ, Hill RA. Skeletal tuberculosis in children in the Western world: 18 new cases with a review of the literature. J Child Orthop 2009;3:319–324
13. Guo LX, Ma YZ, Li HW, Xue HB, Peng W, Luo XB. Variety of ESR and C-reactive protein levels during perioperative period in spinal tuberculosis. [Article in Chinese]. Zhongguo Gu Shang 2010;23:200–202
14. Kumar R, Das RK, Mahapatra AK. Role of interferon gamma release assay in the diagnosis of Pott disease. J Neurosurg Spine 2010;12:462–466
15. Steingart KR, Sohn H, Schiller I, et al. Xpert® MTB/RIF assay for pulmonary tuberculosis and rifampicin resistance in adults. Cochrane Database Syst Rev 2013; 1:CD009593
16. Sharma A, Chhabra HS, Mahajan R, Chabra T, Batra S. Magnetic resonance imaging and GeneXpert: a rapid and accurate diagnostic tool for the management of tuberculosis of the spine. Asian Spine J 2016;10: 850–856
17. Held M, Laubscher M, Zar HJ, Dunn RN. GeneXpert polymerase chain reaction for spinal tuberculosis: an accurate and rapid diagnostic test. Bone Joint J 2014; 96-B:1366–1369
18. Jung NY, Jee WH, Ha KY, Park CK, Byun JY. Discrimination of tuberculous spondylitis from pyogenic spondylitis on MRI. AJR Am J Roentgenol 2004;182: 1405–1410
19. Jain AK, Sreenivasan R, Saini NS, Kumar S, Jain S, Dhammi IK. Magnetic resonance evaluation of tubercular lesion in spine. Int Orthop 2012;36:261–269

9

Drug Therapy for Spinal Tuberculosis

Mathew Varghese

▣ Introduction

Tubercular infection of the spine is an infection of the vertebral elements by *Mycobacterium tuberculosis* or its variants. Like all infections, antimicrobial chemotherapy remains the cornerstone of treatment. The unique microbiological characteristics of the bacteria include a special cell wall that makes it resistant to conventional antibiotics, a slow multiplication rate that necessitates a need for long-term therapy, early development of drug resistance with monotherapy, and the presence of a dormant phase of the bacteria that is unaffected by drugs. All these factors contribute to difficulties in eradicating the bacteria from the site of infection. Chemotherapy of spinal tuberculosis is therefore a challenge due to the special bacterial features, the need for long-term multidrug therapy, and rising the incidence of drug resistance.

▣ History

It is useful to study the history of chemotherapy in order to understand the evolution of treatment regimens and the duration of chemotherapy for tuberculosis (TB). Until the 1940s, there was no drug available for the treatment of TB. The development of streptomycin in 1943 by a team led by Selman Waksman was a

landmark in the treatment of TB. The first trial of streptomycin efficacy, in 1947, was conducted by the Medical Research Council (MRC) of the United Kingdom,[1] which is credited as being the first randomized controlled trial in the world, because it used a statistically based random sampling method.

A second drug, para-aminosalicylic acid (PAS), was evaluated to treat pulmonary TB in Sweden,[2] which led to the MRC's second clinical trial in 1948. The antituberculous properties of isoniazid were observed in 1952. The MRC conducted a further trial of chemotherapy for TB in 1956, in which patients were given chemotherapy for varying lengths of time, from 6 months to 3 years. Introduction of rifampin in 1966 and pyrazinamide in the early 1970s further reduced the relapse rates.

Chemotherapy for osteoarticular TB was based on the experience gained in the treatment of pulmonary TB. Initially, there was apprehension that the antituberculous drugs may not be reaching minimum inhibitory concentration (MIC) levels in the osseous tissues and abscesses from mycobacterial infections. However, studies have shown that MIC levels are reached in the osseous tissues and abscesses. In the tuberculous joints as well as in the cold abscesses, the concentrations were much higher than those considered to have an inhibitory effect on the bacilli in clinical material.[3] In a study on drug concentrations in healing lesions,

Kumar[4] found that the anti-TB drugs penetrated the fibrous tissue surrounding the tuberculous spinal lesions at a therapeutically adequate concentration.

The goals of chemotherapy in TB of the spine are as follows:

- Cure the patient of the infection from mycobacteria.
- Prevent development of drug-resistant TB.
- Prevent development or aid recovery of a neurologic deficit.
- Prevent disability from a mycobacterial infection.
- Prevent relapse of a mycobacterial infection.

The unique nature of the bacilli and the pathogenesis of spinal tubercular infection makes it difficult task to achieve these goals.

Issues in Osteoarticular Tuberculosis

The following subsections discuss the issues peculiar to the nature of infection in spinal TB.

The Nature of Osteoarticular Spinal Tuberculosis

Spinal infection is always a secondary TB and is a paucibacillary disease. The disease evolves slowly, and the degree of destruction of bone depends on multiple factors, from host immunity to virulence of the organism. Clinical features such as pain, swelling, weight loss, fever, and malaise are all nonspecific. Cold abscesses and discharging sinuses, neurologic deficit, and kyphosis may all take time to appear. Neurologic deficit may be the result of active disease or may appear late due to an internal gibbus after healing of the disease. The early radiological manifestation may be completely nonspecific. The radiological response to treatment also is slow, and follow-up radiographs may take months before showing signs of healing. Blood investigations are also nonspecific. All

these features make it difficult for the clinician to decide on the criteria to initiate antitubercular drugs. In endemic zones, a middle path is recommended in which patients are followed up with conservative chemotherapy, and a decision regarding pursuing surgery is based on the specific indications[5]; chemotherapy is continued for the appropriate duration.

End Point of Treatment

The problem in chemotherapy of spinal TB is the assessment of the end point of activity of the disease. Sputum examination in pulmonary TB is a key factor that helps in assessing the response to chemotherapy, whereas in spinal TB, there are no easily available investigations to periodically assess the response to chemotherapy. Currently, a combination of clinical improvements in symptoms, hematological assessment of blood inflammatory markers, and magnetic resonance imaging (MRI) features of vertebral healing are used to assess the healing and to assess the end point of the chemotherapy.

The classic radiographic signs of healing include sclerosis in the previously osteopenic bones, fusion of vertebrae in the case of paradiskal TB, and the filling up or sclerosis of the lytic lesions. However, this process may take a long time. Also, the process of radiological change continues well beyond bacteriological sterility of the lesion.

An MRI with contrast has been used by some surgeons to evaluate the activity of the disease.[6] But MRI can only demonstrate the vascularity or the fluid in the area and not the bacteriological sterilization. The return of normal signal characteristics may take a long time. There could also be paradoxical worsening of lesions during successful TB treatment. This phenomenon is called a paradoxical response or an immune reconstitution inflammatory syndrome (IRIS), and is well known to occur with or without human immunodeficiency virus (HIV) co-infection.[7] So when an MRI is done 2 or 3 months after the start of chemotherapy, it may show an increase in abscess collection. This may lead the surgeon to conclude that the patient is not responding to treatment, whereas this is only an immune response to the tubercular protein. Recent reports on the use of positron emission tomography (PET)/computed tomography (CT) to assess activity of the disease, however, are encouraging. The PET/CT technology enables detailed analysis of changes in individual tuberculous lesions over time and monitoring of the response of these lesions to treatment.[8]

Drug Treatment in Tuberculosis

Drug-Sensitive Tuberculosis Treatment

Chemotherapy initiated in the early stages of the disease will reduce the risks of deformity, neurologic deficit, and disability.

There are three important determinations to make regarding drug treatment for TB:

1. Which drugs?
2. Which regimen?
3. What duration?

Which Drugs?

The World Health Organization (WHO)[9] has classified drugs used in the treatment of TB as follows:

Group 1: first-line oral agents: isoniazid, rifampin, ethambutol, pyrazinamide, and rifabutin
Group 2: injectable agents: kanamycin, amikacin, capreomycin, and streptomycin
Group 3: fluoroquinolones, moxifloxacin, levofloxacin, gatifloxacin, and ofloxacin
Group 4: oral bacteriostatic second-line agents: ethionamide, protionamide, cycloserine, terizidone, and para-aminosalicylic acid
Group 5: agents with unclear efficacy: clofazimine, linezolid, amoxicillin-clavulanate, thiacetazone, clarithromycin, and carbapenems

The various drugs in these groups along with their dosages and key adverse effects are summarized in **Tables 9.1, 9.2, 9.3, 9.4, 9.5.** These groupings have now been reevaluated and modified based on drugs that are effective in multidrug-resistant (MDR) or extensive drug resistant (XDR) TB.[10]

Some of these drugs are bactericidal and some are bacteriostatic; some are effective against intracellular bacteria, and some are active only against extracellular bacteria. Isonia-

Table 9.1 Group 1: First-Line Oral Agents

Drug	Year First Available	Standard Abbreviation for Drug	Per kg Dose (mg)	Two Most Major Side Effects	Major Interaction
Isoniazid (INH)	1952	H	4–6	Hepatitis, peripheral neuritis	Risk of CNS toxicity when given with cycloserine
Rifampin	1963	R	8–12	Hepatitis, orange discoloration of urine	Oral contraceptives, CI with many antiretroviral therapy drugs
Pyrazinamide	1954	Z	20–30	Hepatotoxic, hyperuricemia	Pharmacodynamic synergism with rifampin, decreases effect of probenecid
Ethambutol	1962	E	15–20	Optic neuritis (usually reversible), hypersensitivity	Decreases effects of uricosuric drugs

Abbreviations: CI, contraindicated; CNS, central nervous system.

Table 9.2 Group 2: Injectable Agents

Drug	Year First Available	Standard Abbreviation for Drug	Per kg Dose (mg)	Two Most Major Side Effects	Major Interaction
Streptomycin	1944	S	15	Nephrotoxicity, auditory and vestibular toxicity	↑ risk of nephrotoxicity cyclosporine and cephalosporins; ototoxicity with loop diuretics; hypo-calcemia with bisphosphonates
Kanamycin	1963	Km	15–30	Nephrotoxicity, auditory and vestibular toxicity	↑ risk of nephrotoxicity, with colistin, ototoxicity with loop diuretics, neurotoxic-ity with succinyl choline
Amikacin	1954	Am	15–30	Nephrotoxicity, auditory and vestibular toxicity	↑ risk of nephrotoxicity, cyclosporine, cephalosporins; ototoxicity with loop diuretics; hypo-calcemia with bisphosphonates
Capreomycin	1962	Cm	15–30	Nephrotoxicity, auditory and vestibular toxicity	↑ risk of nephrotoxicity and ototoxicity with aminoglycosides

Table 9.3 Group 3: Fluoroquinolones

Drug	Year First Available	Standard Abbreviation for Drug	Dose (mg)	Two Most Major Side Effects	Major Interaction
Moxifloxacin	1990	Mfx	400 once daily	Arthropathy, arthritis	↑ risk of ventricular arrhythmias with amiodarone, enhances effects of coumarin
Levofloxacin	1996	Lfx	750–1,000 once daily	Gastrointestinal effects, rashes	↑ risk of ventricular arrhythmias with amiodarone, enhances effects of coumarin
Gatifloxacin	1999	Gfx	400 once daily	Hypoglycemia in type 2 diabetes mellitus, dizziness and insomnia	Antacid reduce absorption, ↑ digoxin toxicity, enhances effects of coumarin
Ofloxacin	1980	Ofx	400 twice daily	Arthropathy	Antacids reduce absorption, enhances effects of coumarin

Table 9.4 Group 4: Oral Bacteriostatic Second-Line Agents

Drug	Year First available	Standard Abbreviation for Drug	Per kg Dose (mg)	Two Most Major Side Effects	Major Interaction
Ethionamide	1956	Eto	15–20 in 2–3 divided doses	Hepatotoxicity, hypothyroidism	Enhanced toxic effects with alcohol, ↑ toxic effects of cycloserine
Protionamide		Pto	15–20	Gastrointestinal side effects, hypothyroidism	↑ risk of neurotoxicity with cycloserine, ↑ risk of hepatotoxicity with rifampin
Cycloserine	1954	Cs	10–20	Psychosis, depression	↑ risk of convulsions with alcohol, ↑ risk of CNS toxicity with INH
Terizidone		Trd	10–20	Psychosis, depression (suicidal)	
p-Amino salicylic acid	1902	PAS	200–300	Hepatotoxicity, hypothyroidism	Prothionamide ↑ increased risk of side effects, ↓ absorption of digoxin

zid, rifampin, streptomycin, and ethambutol act on extracellular rapidly multiplying ($< 10^8$) bacteria. Rifampin acts on extracellular slowly multiplying ($< 10^5$) bacteria also. Pyrazinamide acts on both intra- and extracellular bacteria in an acidic environment ($< 10^5$). Lesions may also harbor bacteria that are dormant and not multiplying at all. As yet there are no drugs available to eliminate these bacteria.

In the early active phase of the disease, the bacteria are rapidly multiplying and their numbers are large. Treatment at this intensive phase entails using drugs that are effective against both intra- and extracellular bacteria. A drug such as pyrazinamide is mainly effective in an acidic medium and is most effective in the first 2 months of treatment. There is no additional advantage to continuing pyrazinamide beyond the first 2 months.[11] The 5-year total relapse rates for patients with drug-susceptible strains were 3.4% for a pyrazinamide series compared with 10.3% for a non-pyrazinamide series ($p < 0.001$).[11] This highlights the importance of including pyrazinamide in the combinations used.

Which Regimen?

Chemotherapeutic drug regimens are based on the experience gained in the treatment of pulmonary TB.[12] Inappropriate regimens and arbitrary changes of drugs contribute to the development of drug resistance. The development of drug resistance with single drug therapy was recognized early, during the first trials of streptomycin. In a study evaluating prescription patterns among private practitioners, Udwadia et al[13] found that only six of 106 responding practitioners wrote a prescription with the correct drug regimen. The 106 doctors prescribed 63 different drug regimens. This highlights the importance of publishing, and distributing to practitioners, the appropriate drug protocols for TB treatment.

Table 9.5 Group 5: Agents with Unclear Efficacy

Drug	Year First Available	Standard Abbreviation for Drug	Dose (mg)	Major Side Effects	Major Interaction
Clofazimine	1954	Cfz	100 once daily	Skin, retina, cornea urine, discoloration, Gastrointestinal side effects	Bedaquiline and fluoroquinolones- ↑ risk of prolong QTc
Linezolid	2000	Lzd	600 (10 mg/kg)	Myelosuppression, thrombocytopenia	↑ serum level with clarithromycin, avoid tyramine-rich foods
Amoxicillin-clavulanate	1984	Amx-Clv	2,000/125 twice daily	Gastrointestinal effects, rashes	Increased INR in patients taking coumarin
Thioacetazone	1951	T	150 once daily	Hepatotoxicity, neutropenia, anemia, thrombocytopenia	Streptomycin. possibly increased ototoxicity
Clarithromycin	1980		500 twice daily	Gastrointestinal effects, rashes, hepatotoxicity	Colchicine- ↑ renal, hepatic toxicity in impairment, ↑ risk of myopathy with statins
Carbapenems	1985	Imipenem-Ipm Meropenem-Mpm	Different doses for different drugs	Gastrointestinal effects, rashes, DRESS syndrome	↓ effect of BCG, typhoid, cholera vaccines, ↓ effect valproate

Note: Data for these table have been collected from multiple sources.
Abbreviations: BCG, Bacille Calmette-Guerin; DRESS, drug reaction with eosinophilia and systemic symptoms; INR, international normalized ratio.

Natural drug resistance in *M. tuberculosis* is as low as 10^{-3} to 10^{-8} for one drug, 10^{-12} to 10^{-14} for two drugs, and 10^{-18} to 10^{-20} for three drugs.[14] When three or more drugs are utilized together for the treatment of TB, the risk of acquiring drug resistance is negligible.

For drug-sensitive tubercular infection, the standard regimen recommended by the WHO is isoniazid (isonicotinic acid hydrazide, INH), rifampin (RIF), pyrazinamide (PZA), and ethambutol (EMB) for 2 months followed by a continuation phase of 4 months of INH and RIF.[9,15] The Centers for Disease Control and Prevention (CDC) also recommends the same regimen for treating adults with TB.[16] All the other drugs listed in the groups are for special situations, such as MDR or XDR TB or drug allergy. By and large, there is no controversy on the choice of drugs for bone and joint TB.

What Duration?

All regimens have an intensive phase and a continuation phase. In drug-sensitive TB, the intensive phase lasts 2 months, and the continuation phase may vary from 4 months to 8 to

10 months. It is the killing dynamics of the intracellular *M. tuberculosis* bacterial population that predominantly determines the treatment duration.[17] The long duration of chemotherapy naturally has inherent problems, such as lack of compliance and treatment failure.[18] The introduction of short-term chemotherapy, therefore, was important for improving adherence to treatment regimens. Trials by the MRC of the UK showed that shorter courses could also be effective without increasing the relapse rates. The MRC found that short-course regimens based on isoniazid and rifampin are as effective as 18-month regimens; ambulatory chemotherapy with these regimens should now be the standard management of uncomplicated spinal TB.[19] The radiological changes continue to evolve from lysis, to gradually increasing bone density and sclerosis, to fusion of contiguous vertebrae in paradiskal disease.

Directly observed treatment, short course (DOTS) was introduced by the WHO in 1991 to ensure adherence to treatment protocols by providing supervised treatment by a health care worker.[20] DOTS treatment administered by a health care worker on alternate days or every third day was based on the behavior of the *M. tuberculosis* bacteria on exposure to antitubercular drugs. Bacteria in a culture of *M. tuberculosis* exposed for 24 hours to an antitubercular drug do not start multiplying even after the drug is washed away. The number of bacteria continues to fall for some time. The period when the drug is not available and before the organism starts multiplying is called the lag phase.[21] Existence of the lag phase enables implementing an intermittent therapy regimen without the risk of the patient's developing drug resistance. That was the basis of intermittent DOTS, which enabled the health care worker to visit the patient with pulmonary TB not every day but every other day or every third day to supervise the treatment. DOTS was just a mechanism of delivering short-course chemotherapy with a more effective implementation of policy.[22] DOTS centers were set up in many countries by departments of health in consultation with the WHO to reduce the dropout rate of patients on treatment and to reduce the development of drug-resistant TB. Currently, the WHO defines DOTS treatment as a patient taking medications in real time under the observation of a health care worker, or even just a friend, a relative, or another layperson who functions as a treatment supervisor or supporter.[15]

Van Loenhout-Rooyackers et al,[23] in a review of the literature, found a 0% relapse rate after 6 months of HRZ [isoniazid (H), rifampin (R), pyrazinamide (Z)] treatment. Researchers have even tried ultra-short regimens in conjunction with thorough focal debridement, bone grafting, and internal fixation, and they found the effectiveness to be similar to that of standard chemotherapy in the treatment of spinal TB. However, this is not recommended as a standard treatment guideline.[24]

The CDC recommends that pulmonary and extrapulmonary disease should be treated with the same regimen.[16] The UK's National Institutes for Clinical Excellence guidelines (2016) also recommend that patients with active TB without central nervous system involvement (meningitis) be treated with HRZE [isoniazid (H), rifampin (R), pyrazinamide (Z), and ethambutol (E)] for 2 months and then with isoniazid and rifampin for a further 4 months. The treatment regimen should be modified based on drug susceptibility testing.[25] Although there is no supporting evidence, some experts favor a 9-month duration of treatment because of the difficulties in assessing the treatment response. In the setting of extensive orthopedic hardware, some experts extend the duration of treatment further to 12 months.[16] Uncomplicated cases of spinal TB are managed with medical rather than surgical treatment.

Fig. 9.1 shows the case of a 51-year-old man with T6-T7 tuberculosis that was managed with standard antitubercular chemotherapy. The posttreatment image of the patient shows complete resolution of the lesion (**Fig. 9.1b**). The patient had no neurologic deficit.

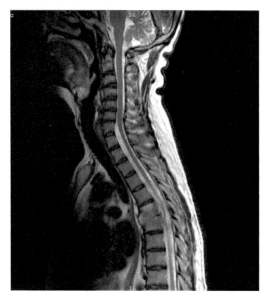
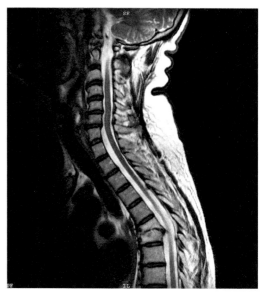

a   b

Fig. 9.1 **(a)** A 51-year-old man patient with T6-T7 tuberculosis (TB) managed with standard antitubercular chemotherapy. **(b)** Posttreatment image shows complete resolution. The patient had no neurologic deficit.

Multidrug-Resistant Tuberculosis

The careless overuse of antibiotics has created a situation in which the treatment of *M. tuberculosis* first encountered mono-drug resistance, then multidrug resistance (MDR), then extensive drug resistance (XDR), and eventually totally drug resistance (TDR), because of the sequential accumulation of resistance mutations.[26] The term MDR is used if mycobacteria exhibit resistance to both isoniazid and rifampin.

Clinical suspicion is important in diagnosing MDR TB, but the diagnosis must be based on bacteriological/molecular testing, as MDR TB is a bacteriological diagnosis and not a clinical diagnosis. Patients at high risk of MDR TB are those who have had drug treatment for TB earlier, or who are in social contact with patients in treatment for MDR or XDR TB. Health care workers who are likely to come into contact with patients in treatment for TB or persons coming from areas where the WHO reports show greater than 5% prevalence of MDR TB are also at risk. Co-infection with HIV may also make a patient vulnerable to MDR and XDR TB. Irrespective of the epidemic setting, the WHO now recommends HIV testing for patients of all ages who present with signs or symptoms that suggest TB, whether TB is suspected or already confirmed.[15] Specimens for culture and drug susceptibility testing (DST) should be obtained from all previously treated TB patients at or before the start of treatment. DST should be performed for at least isoniazid and rifampin.[9]

In spinal TB, obtaining a sample for molecular diagnostics is difficult, so if the clinical and imaging modalities are highly suspicious, then empirical drug therapy could be started. But with the increasing incidence of drug-resistant TB, every effort should be made to procure a specimen for culture and molecular diagnostics before starting treatment. If there is a paraspinal abscess or psoas abscess, pus must be aspirated for testing. Even in the absence of any pus collection, a specimen for culture and molecular tests must be obtained under image intensifier or CT scan guidance.

Treatment of MDR TB is challenging, as the combination drugs that are available are more toxic, and many need to be given parenterally for a longer period. It is not recommended to add a single drug to a failing drug regimen—the so-called addition syndrome.[27] Once resistance has developed, the DOTS strategy can paradoxically exacerbate the problem—the so-called the amplifier effect of short course chemotherapy.[28] It is advisable to seek the help of an infectious disease specialist in cases of MDR and XDR.

At least four second-line anti-TB drugs likely to be effective should be included in the MDR regimen. All regimens should include a new-generation fluoroquinolone such as levofloxacin or moxifloxacin.[29]

Revised Grouping of Drugs

The WHO has regrouped drugs used in MDR TB based on newer available evidence available[10]:

Group A: levofloxacin, moxifloxacin, gatifloxacin

Group B: amikacin, capreomycin, kanamycin (streptomycin)

Group C: ethionamide (or prothionamide), cycloserine (or terizidone), linezolid, clofazimine

Group D1: pyrazinamide ethambutol high-dose isoniazid

Group D2: bedaquiline, delamanid

Group D3: p-aminosalicylic acid, imipenem-cilastatin, meropenem, amoxicillin-clavulanate, thioacetazone

In MDR TB, at least five effective TB drugs must be given during the intensive phase, including pyrazinamide, and four core second-line TB drugs, one from group A, one from group B, and at least two from group C.[28]

Fig. 9.2 shows the case of an 18-year-old man with MDR TB of the T7-T8 vertebrae on HRZE treatment for 2 months. Culture and DST show resistance to INH and rifampin. The patient was started on second-line antitubercular drugs (6 months: tab levofloxacin, inj. kanamycin, inj. ethionamide inj. cycloserine, tab pyrazinamide, and tab ethambutol; 12 months: tab levofloxacin, inj. ethionamide, inj. cycloserine, and tab ethambutol). Imaging performed at the end of 1 year still showed some residual

infection (**Fig. 9.2b**). At 18 months, resolution of the soft tissue abscess and healing of the infection was noted on T2-weighted imaging (**Fig. 9.2c**).

Extensively Drug-Resistant Tuberculosis

In 2006, the term *extensively drug-resistant TB* (XDR TB) was coined to describe strains of MDR TB resistant to fluoroquinolones and at least one second-line injectable drugs (capreomycin, kanamycin, and amikacin).[28] This again is based on drug sensitivity testing and hence is a laboratory diagnosis. Therefore, every attempt must be made to obtain samples for a bacteriological diagnosis. All patients diagnosed with MDR TB should be tested for XDR TB. This includes testing for resistance to the three second-line injectable drugs (kanamycin, amikacin, and capreomycin) and at least one fluoroquinolone.[28] Treatment must be customized on a case-by-case basis.

Two additional drugs that are showing promise are bedaquiline and delamanid.[30] They are presently classified as group D2,[10] and their use is recommended in adults with XDR for a maximum of 6 months. Both are cardiotoxic and increase the QT interval.[30] Most of the experience gained in MDR and XDR TB is from the treatment of pulmonary TB, with very few reports on spinal TB .[27,31] Radiographs and MRI of a 19-year-old student nurse without neurologic deficit show a tuberculous spine at C5-C6 (**Fig. 9.3a,b**). The patient underwent surgery to decompress the abscess and stabilize the spine. Immediate and 3 weeks postoperative radiographs show the implant backing out and pus reforming (**Fig. 9.3c,d**). Pus culture revealed XDR TB resistant to all first-line drugs, kanamycin, ethionamide, amikacin, PAS, and fluoroquinolones. Hence, patient was started on claribid, moxifloxacin, cycloserine, isoniazid, thiacetazone, and injection amikacin for 2 years. The posttreatment 3-year follow-up radiograph shows complete resolution of the disease and the patient's full recovery (**Fig. 9.3e**).

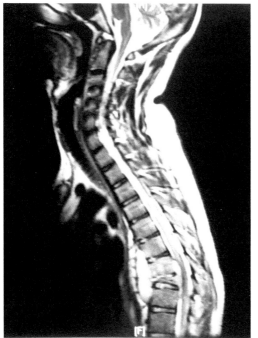

a

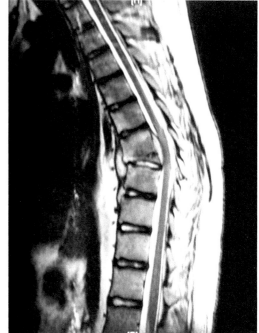

b

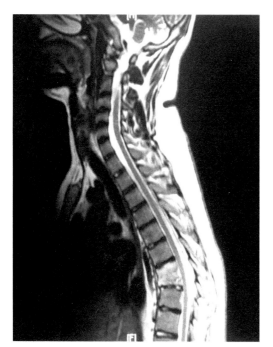

c

Fig. 9.2 An 18-year-old man presents with multidrug-resistant (MDR) TB of the T7-T8 vertebrae. He has been on HRZE [isoniazid (H), rifampin (R), pyrazinamide (Z), and ethambutol (E)] for 2 months. **(a)** Culture and drug susceptibility testing (DST) show resistance to isoniazid and rifampin. Patient was started on second-line antitubercular drugs: (6 months: tab levofloxacin, inj. kanamycin, inj. ethionamide, inj. cycloserine, tab pyrazinamide, and tab ethambutol; 12 months: tab levofloxacin, inj. ethionamide, inj. cycloserine, and tab ethambutol). **(b)** Imaging performed at the end of 1 year still shows some residual infection. **(c)** At 18 months, resolution of soft tissue abscess and healing of infection on a T2-weighted image is noted.

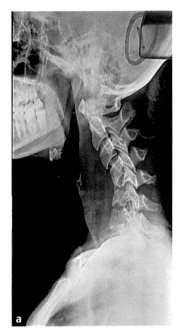

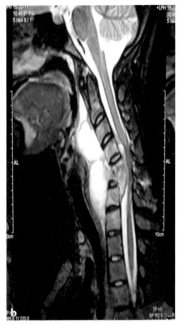

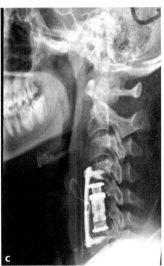

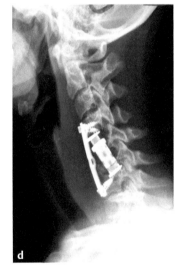

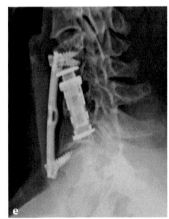

Fig. 9.3 A 19-year-old student nurse presents with tuberculous spine at C5-C6 without neurologic deficit. **(a)** Radiograph. **(b)** Magnetic resonance imaging (MRI). The patient underwent surgery to decompress the abscess and stabilize the spine. **(c)** Immediate and **(d)** 3 weeks postoperative radiographs show the implant backing out and pus reforming. Pus culture revealed XDR TB resistant to all first-line drugs, kanamycin, ethionamide, amikacin, PAS, and fluoroquinolones. Hence, the patient was started on claribid, moxifloxacin, cycloserine, isoniazid, thiacetazone, and injection amikacin for 2 years. **(e)** Posttreatment 3-year follow-up radiograph after completion of treatment shows complete resolution of the disease and full recovery of the patient.

Chapter Summary

Treatment of spinal TB is essentially medical management of a bacterial infection, with drug treatment as its cornerstone. The unique characteristics of *Mycobacterium*—the cell wall, the slow multiplication time and ability to rapidly mutate to drug resistant forms with a persistent dormant state, and the absence of a clear end point for treatment—render it a difficult infection to treat. To avoid relapses and the development of drug-resistant TB, it is important to have clear protocols for treatment. The standard regimen for DST is to have 2 months of intensive treatment with HRZE and 6 to 9 (or even 12) months of HR depending on the clinical response to treatment. In cases with an inadequate response to treatment, never add a single drug in the hope of tackling drug resistance. MDR and XDR infections are bacteriological diagnoses, and every effort must be made to acquire a pus specimen for culture as well as molecular diagnostics before starting treatment. Treatment of MDR or XDR is a special situation that requires consulting a specialist.

Pearls

♦ Treatment of spinal TB is essentially medical, with drug treatment in two phases—an intensive phase and a continuation phase.

♦ In all patients, especially those at risk of MDR or XDR TB, attempts must be made to obtain a specimen for culture and drug sensitivity before starting therapy.

♦ Four drugs (HRZE) are essential in the intensive phase and at least two drugs (HR) in the continuation phase. The addition of ethambutol to the continuation phase has been recommended recently.

♦ Short-course therapy is effective in spinal TB, but the duration should be titrated by the response to treatment. Although 6 months would be adequate in most patients, it may be extended to 9 or 12 months in those who do not show complete healing.

♦ A daily drug regimen is recommended in spinal TB.

Pitfalls

♦ MRI is unreliable for assessing the response to treatment in the early phases of disease. An exaggerated immune response can result in an increase in the abscess size in the early stages, paradoxically.

♦ In patients not responding to standard chemotherapy, a single drug should not be added to a failing regimen.

♦ A repeat tissue culture and drug sensitivity testing (DST) should be performed to diagnose MDR and XDR infections.

♦ Drug resistance is an emerging problem, and hence appropriate dosing and duration should be strictly followed.

♦ Drug treatment for MDR and XDR must be based on DST. Because it involves multiple drugs with higher adverse effects, an infectious disease specialist must be consulted for treating MDR and XDR TB.

References

Five Must-Read References

1. Leeming-Latham C. Unravelling the "tangled web": chemotherapy for tuberculosis in Britain, 1940–70 the William Bynum prize essay. Med Hist 2015;59: 156–176

2. Lehmann J. The treatment of tuberculosis in Sweden with para-aminosalicylic acid: a review. Dis Chest 1949;16:684–703, illust

3. Tuli SM, Kumar K, Sen PC. Penetration of antitubercular drugs in clinical osteoarticular tubercular lesions. Acta Orthop Scand 1977;48:362–368

4. Kumar K. The penetration of drugs into the lesions of spinal tuberculosis. Int Orthop 1992;16:67–68 (SICOT)

5. Tuli SM. Results of treatment of spinal tuberculosis by "middle-path" regime. J Bone Joint Surg Br 1975; 57:13–23

6. Jain AK, Srivastava A, Saini NS, Dhammi IK, Sreenivasan R, Kumar S. Efficacy of extended DOTS category I chemotherapy in spinal tuberculosis based on MRI-based healed status. Indian J Orthop 2012;46: 633–639

7. Breen RA, Smith CJ, Bettinson H, et al. Paradoxical reactions during tuberculosis treatment in patients with and without HIV co-infection. Thorax 2004; 59:704–707

8. Barry CE III, Boshoff HI, Dartois V, et al. The spectrum of latent tuberculosis: rethinking the biology and intervention strategies. Nat Rev Microbiol 2009;7: 845–855

9. World Health Organization (WHO). Treatment of Tuberculosis: Guidelines, 4th ed. Geneva: World Health Organization; 2010

10. World Health Organization (WHO). WHO Treatment guidelines for drug-resistant tuberculosis—2016 update. Geneva: World Health Organization; 2016

11. Five year follow up of a controlled trial of five six month regimens of chemotherapy for pulmonary tuberculosis. Hong Kong Chest Service/British Medical Research Council. Am Rev Respir Dis 1987;136: 139–1342

12. Fox W, Ellard GA, Mitchison DA. Studies on the treatment of tuberculosis undertaken by the British Medical Research Council tuberculosis units, 1946–1986, with relevant subsequent publications. Int J Tuberc Lung Dis 1999;3(10, Suppl 2):S231–S279

13. Udwadia ZF, Pinto LM, Uplekar MW. Tuberculosis management by private practitioners in Mumbai, India: has anything changed in two decades? PLoS One 2010;5:e12023

14. Shimao T. Drug resistance in tuberculosis control. Tubercle 1987;68(2, Suppl):5–18

15. World Health Organization (WHO). Treatment of Tuberculosis guidelines for treatment of drug-susceptible tuberculosis and patient care 2017 update. Geneva: World Health Organization; 2017

16. Nahid P, Dorman SE, Alipanah N, et al. American Thoracic Society/Centers for Disease Control and Prevention/Infectious Diseases Society of America Clinical Practice Guidelines: Treatment of Drug-Susceptible Tuberculosis. Clinical infectious diseases advance access. Clin Infect Dis 2016;63:e147–e195.

17. Aljayyoussin G, Jenkins VA, Sharma R, et al. Pharmacokinetic-pharmacodynamic modelling of intracellular Mycobacterium tuberculosis growth and kill rates is predictive of clinical treatment duration. J Thorac Dis 2017;9:2093–2101

18. Sarkar S. An overview of tuberculosis chemotherapy: a literature review. J Pharm Sci 2011;14:148–161

19. Medical Research Council. A 15-year assessment of controlled trials of the management of tuberculosis of the spine in Korea and Hong Kong. Thirteenth Report of the Medical Research Council Working Party on Tuberculosis of the Spine. J Bone Joint Surg Br 1998;80:456–462

20. What is DOTS? A guide to understanding the WHO-recommended TB control strategy known as DOTS. http://apps.who.int/iris/bitstream/10665/65979/1/WHO_CDS_CPC_TB_99.270.pdf

21. Dickinson JM, Mitchison DA. In vitro studies on the choice of drugs for intermittent chemotherapy of tuberculosis. Tubercle 1966;47:370–380

22. Weis SE, Slocum PC, Blais FX, et al. The effect of directly observed therapy on the rates of drug resistance and relapse in tuberculosis. N Engl J Med 1994; 330:1179–1184

23. van Loenhout-Rooyackers JH, Verbeek ALM, Jutte PC. Chemotherapeutic treatment for spinal tuberculosis. Int J Tuberc Lung Dis 2002;6:259–265

24. Wang Z, Shi J, Geng G, Qiu H. Ultra-short-course chemotherapy for spinal tuberculosis: five years of observation. Eur Spine J 2013;22:274–281

25. National Institutes for Clinical Excellence (NICE). Guidelines, 2016. https://www.nice.org.uk/guidance/ng33/chapter/recommendations#diagnosing-extrapulmonary-tb-in-all-age-groups

26. Nguyen L. Antibiotic resistance mechanisms in M. tuberculosis: an update. Arch Toxicol 2016;90:1585–1604

27. Mohan K, Rawall S, Pawar UM, et al. Drug resistance patterns in 111 cases of drug-resistant tuberculosis spine. Eur Spine J 2013;22(Suppl 4):647–652

28. Seung KJ, Keshavjee S, Rich ML. Multi drug resistant tuberculosis and extensively drug resistant tuberculosis. Cold Spring Harb Perspect Med 2015;5:a017863

29. Johnson JL, Hadad DJ, Boom WH, et al. Early and extended early bactericidal activity of levofloxacin, gatifloxacin and moxifloxacin in pulmonary tuberculosis. Int J Tuberc Lung Dis 2006;10:605–612

30. D'Ambrosio L, Centis R, Tiberi S, et al. Delamanid and bedaquiline to treat multidrug-resistant and extensively drug-resistant tuberculosis in children: a systematic review. J Thorac Dis 2017;9:2093–2101

31. Pawar UM, Kundnani V, Agashe V, Nene A, Nene A. Multidrug-resistant tuberculosis of the spine—is it the beginning of the end? A study of 25 culture proven multidrug-resistant tuberculosis spine patients. Spine 2009;34:E806–E810

10

Surgical Management of Spinal Tuberculosis

Ajoy Prasad Shetty, Rishi M. Kanna, and S. Rajasekaran

Introduction

Early diagnosis along with effective multidrug antituberculous chemotherapy has revolutionized the treatment of spinal tuberculosis (TB) and has obviated the need for surgery in the majority of patients. However, additional surgical intervention may be necessary in those who are diagnosed or present late, as chemotherapy alone may not be able to reverse the consequences of disk and vertebral destruction. Spinal TB primarily affects the anterior column of the spine, and progressive vertebral destruction with collapse may result in significant kyphosis and neurological deficit, thus necessitating surgery. The goals of surgery are to ensure adequate decompression, debridement, maintenance, and reinforcement of stability and correcting the deformity or halting the progress of deformity.

Historical Perspective and Evolution of Treatment

Historically, Hibbs in 1911 and Albee in 1913 advocated posterior fusion to prevent further progression of deformity with unpredictable results. Capener and later Wilkinson and Seddon demonstrated the efficacy of debridement by the costotransversectomy approach, which was termed anterolateral rachitomy.[1] Hodgson

and Stock[2] in 1956 popularized the Hong Kong procedure, which not only revolutionized the surgical management of spinal TB but also paved the way for the anterior approach for other spinal pathologies, too. The Hong Kong procedure was considered the gold standard approach; it included radical debridement of the lesion and anterior interbody fusion with tricortical iliac or fibular strut grafts through an anterior approach. Severe neurologic deficit and significant kyphosis have always been considered as definitive indications for surgery.

To identify the role of surgery in patients without a neurologic deficit, the British Medical Research Council (MRC) conducted a series of prospective multicenter randomized clinical trials that compared the results of chemotherapy alone (an ambulatory regimen of rifampin and isoniazid) with debridement alone and with radical debridement and anterior spinal fusion together. Both short- and long-term findings indicated that all the three treatments achieved similarly favorable clinical results.[3] The favorable status was defined as no evidence of central nervous system involvement, no sinus or clinically evident abscess, no radiological evidence of disease activity, and no restriction of normal physical activity. The major shortcoming of the study was that it did not assess spinal deformity (kyphosis). However, careful evaluation of the short-term results revealed faster resolution of abscess and bony union with the Hong Kong procedure. This advantage was retained in the long-term results, with data showing minimal deformity and maintained sagittal alignment. In contrast, patients treated with chemotherapy and debridement showed relapse of sinuses and recurrence of cold abscesses and worsening of kyphotic deformity. In about 5% of the conservatively treated patients, there was a significant increase of kyphosis from 51 to 70 degrees.[4] The MRC trials also demonstrated resolution of cold abscesses with chemotherapy alone, and hence surgical drainage of cold abscesses is no longer recommended, unless they present with pressure effects.

The use of instrumentation became popular following the work of Oga et al,[5] who showed that tubercle bacilli, unlike pyogenic organisms, neither adhere to metal nor form any biofilm. With the advent of better instrumentation techniques, surgical treatment has yielded better results in terms of early ambulation, good disease clearance, and prevention of progression of deformity. The use of titanium implants enables healing of the disease to be assessed through postoperative imaging with computed tomography (CT) or magnetic resonance imaging (MRI). Although the anterior approach has been traditionally popular, the recent trend is for posterior approach–based spinal stabilization and decompression with or without global reconstruction, especially in the thoracic and lumbar spine. Modern posterior spinal instrumentation systems enable the safe correction of deformity, spinal fusion, and anterior reconstruction of vertebral defects without many complications. In the cervical spine, anterior debridement, reconstruction, and stabilization remain popular.

General Principles of Surgical Management

The advantages of surgical treatment are that it aids in histological confirmation of the diagnosis; decreases the disease burden; enhances the healing, correction, and prevention of spinal deformity; reduces the rate of recurrence; and promotes early neurologic recovery.

The five basic principles of surgical management of spinal TB are debridement, decompression of the spinal canal, correction of deformity, reconstruction of the anterior defect, and spinal stabilization. Depending on the severity of the bone destruction, kyphosis, and neurologic deficit, the surgery may include all or some of the five components.[6] Drainage of the cold abscess is rarely indicated, as anti-TB drugs can effectively resolve it in most cases. Notable indications for abscess drainage include respiratory distress or dysphagia due to a large cervical paravertebral abscess, and pseudo–hip flexion deformity due to a large psoas abscess or an abscess that has tracked into the subcutaneous plane with imminent rupture. Whenever feasible, drainage of the cold abscess by ultrasound guidance is preferred.

Tuberculosis of the spine can be classified based on the vertebral and disk space destruction as pauci-segment or multi-segment disease. Pauci-segment or pauci-level disease is considered to be present when the involvement is limited to two adjoining vertebrae and the intervening disk. Multisegment disease involves more than two vertebral bodies and intervertebral disks and is associated with significant instability and deformity. Multisegment disease can be contiguous or noncontiguous. This classification can guide the surgical treatment with regard to approach, aggressiveness of debridement, and extent of instrumentation.

Debridement and Decompression

A typical surgical procedure for spinal tuberculosis involves debridement of the tuberculous focus—caseous material, granulation tissue, and sequestrated bone up to the posterior longitudinal ligament through an anterior approach. Debridement is extended proximally and distally until the bleeding cancellous bone is exposed from the cephalad and caudal vertebrae. In cases with destruction extending up to the upper or lower end plate, an extensive debridement involving removal of the disks above and below may be necessary. Experimental studies have shown that the concentrations of antitubercular drugs varied greatly in different tissues in spinal TB, and the least concentration and penetration of the drug was noted in the sclerotic focus, thus advocating its removal.[7]

Debridement alone does not the prevent the progression of the deformity nor does it improve healing. Adequate debridement followed by interbody fusion and surgical stabilization relieves pain, improves neurologic function, and prevents deformity. It can be performed either by an anterior approach or by a posterior transfacetal, transpedicular, or costotransversectomy approach.

Reconstruction of the Anterior Defect

The reconstruction of the anterior defect can be performed with autografts, structural allografts, or titanium cages. Iliac crest grafts or ribs are preferred in smaller defects, whereas fibular grafts or tibial grafts are suitable options in larger defects. Autografts should be preferably tricortical autografts, as they provide structural support along with osteogenic potential. In larger defects, a high risk of graft failure has been reported in uninstrumented fusion as the bone tends to be invaded by the creeping substitution process, leading to collapse in the initial stage of remodeling of cortical bone. The use of only cancellous graft or a local autogenous graft along with transpedicular instrumentation could be an option in the lumbar spine. Recently, the trend is to use a titanium cage, as it provides strong mechanical support, enables packing with corticocancellous graft, and minimizes the risk of dislodgment. The use of cages avoids the morbidity of graft harvesting and the loss of strength of strut graft during its resorption phase. Titanium cages can be mesh cages, interbody cages, or expandable cages.[8] Titanium cages grab on to vertebral bone, and settling occurs on vertical loading, providing stability to the cage.

Deformity Correction

The development of kyphosis is the rule in spinal tuberculosis, and it is directly proportional to the destruction of the disk space and vertebral body. In patients treated conservatively, irrespective of the disease severity, it was ob-

served that there was a mean increase of spine deformity by 15 degrees, and at the end of treatment 3 to 5% of patients have a final deformity of more than 60 degrees. Hence, it is important to identify the risk factors leading to the development of severe kyphotic deformity and to surgically treat them in the active phase.[9] The kyphotic deformity during the active stages is usually flexible, and surgical correction of the deformity can be achieved by debridement, reconstruction of the defect, and instrumentation along with anti-TB chemotherapy.

Instrumentation

Spinal instrumentation helps to enhance stability, minimize graft dislodgment, correct deformity, and enable early mobilization and rehabilitation of patients. Additional benefits include providing immediate relief from the instability pain and enabling neurologic recovery. Lee et al[10] and Broner et al[11] reported that the immobilization effect achieved by the instrumentation might also suppress infection and provide a stable environment that can prevent TB recurrence. *Mycobacterium tuberculosis* has less affinity to adhere to biomaterial, and thus the use of titanium implants, which have an active oxide surface, renders less adherence compared with stainless steel implants, making their use safe in the presence of active infection.[5] The levels of instrumentation depend on the site of the lesion, the quality of the bone, and the surgical plan. Ideally, it is preferable to apply fixation at least two levels above and below the lesion. However, in the lumbar spine, in the presence of a rigid anterior interbody construct, one level of fixation above and below the lesion can be adequate. The extent of the spinal instrumentation can be minimized by introducing screws in the upper involved pedicle of the superior vertebral body in paucisegment disease.

Indications of Surgery in Spinal Tuberculosis

Uncomplicated spinal TB is a medical disease, and it can be effectively managed by chemotherapy alone; surgical intervention may be needed in relatively few cases. However, in those cases complicated with TB (gross neurologic deficit, instability, deformity, unresponsive to medical therapy), it is advised that a combination of medical therapy and surgery be used to yield optimum results. Neurologic deficit, especially if it is severe or progressively worsening, and bowel and bladder incontinence are considered absolute indications for surgery. The presence of a stable, nonprogressive neurologic deficit is not an absolute indication for surgery in active spinal TB, as chemotherapy improves the neurologic outcome.[1,2] Tuli[1] introduced a middle-path regimen, wherein he treated neurologic deficit patients initially with bed rest and antituberculous chemotherapy. Surgery was considered only if there was further deterioration of a partial neurologic deficit or if there was no improvement after 3 to 4 weeks. Adding to this regimen, Jain and Kumar,[12] in an MRI-based study, found that cold abscesses causing neurologic deficit resolved with conservative treatment, and for those caused by bony compression and granulation tissue, surgical intervention was necessary. Conservative treatment of patients with a neurologic deficit, although successful, takes more time for neurologic recovery and for the patient to become ambulant. Hence, it would be prudent to consider early surgical decompression and fusion to enable more rapid resolution of the neurologic deficit and an earlier return to normal activity. Surgery is also indicated in multilevel contiguous or noncontiguous disease, pan-vertebral disease, kyphosis greater than 30 degrees, and junctional areas, as they are subjected to a high risk of biomechanical stress and instability.

Rajasekaran[13] described the radiographic "spine-at-risk" signs in pediatric patients that predict the likelihood of developing progressive deformity. These signs, which appear early in the disease, include facet dislocation, retropulsion of the diseased fragments, lateral vertebral translation, and toppling of the superior vertebra. Rajasekaran proposed calculating an instability score; a score of more than 2 indicated disruption of the posterior facet and is an indication for the surgery. These signs can help identify patients who are at risk for deformity

---

Box 10.1 Surgical Indications in Spinal Tuberculosis

- ◆ **Neurologic deficit**
  - Severe neurologic deficit at presentation
  - Rapidly worsening deficits
  - New onset or deterioration of deficits during chemotherapy
  - Unimproved deficits after 6 to 8 weeks of chemotherapy
- ◆ **Spinal instability**
  - Pan-vertebral disease
  - Loss of one vertebral body in the thoracic spine or 1.5 vertebral bodies in the lumbar spine
  - Initial kyphosis of 30 degrees
  - "Spine-at-risk" signs in a child
  - Posterior neural arch lesion with pedicular destruction
  - Axial pain due to instability
- ◆ **Response to chemotherapy**
  - Lack of clinical response after 6 weeks of chemotherapy
  - Recurrence of disease despite chemotherapy
- ◆ **Late deformity**
  - Severe kyphosis with late-onset neurologic deficits

---

progression of more than 30 degrees and a final deformity of over 60 degrees. Rajasekaran and Shanmugasundaram[14] advocated surgery for adults with loss of three fourths of a thoracic or thoracolumbar vertebra, or loss of one lumbar vertebra, aiming for a final kyphosis of no more than 30 degrees. In patients with a doubtful diagnosis, persistent pain, and no response to chemotherapy, surgery is indicated. The indications for surgery are summarized in **Box 10.1**.

Surgical Approach

A single surgical technique cannot be applied universally to all patients. Factors that are taken into consideration when deciding on the specific surgical approach are the age of the patient, the location of the bony lesion, the presence of medical comorbidities, the degree of kyphosis, the region of the spine involved, and the experience and preference of the surgeon. Although anterior approaches are preferred, as they enable thorough evacuation of all infected tissue, the recent trend is for an all-posterior global reconstruction, especially in the thoracic and lumbar spine. Irrespective of the approach used, it is mandatory that the tissue should be sent to the lab for a histopathology evaluation, culture sensitivity, and GeneXpert study.

Anterior Approach

The anterior approach provides direct access to the disease pathology and is ideal for debriding and reconstructing the defect. The anterior approach to the thoracic spine includes the anterolateral extrapleural approach and the transpleural anterior approach popularized by Hodgson et al. The anterior approach involves debridement of the tuberculous focus with removal of the diseased vertebrae, posterior longitudinal ligament (PLL), and adjacent disk spaces until bleeding healthy bone is reached, followed by performing an anterior fusion using a rib graft or a tricortical iliac crest graft. MRC trials have conclusively shown that the Hong Kong operation produced faster bony fusion, less kyphotic deformity, and decreased disease recurrence. The addition of anterior fixation devices has helped to enhance stability, minimize graft displacement, prevent loss of kyphosis, and facilitate early mobilization. In cases with large defects spanning over two or three vertebral bodies without instrumentation, increased risks of graft slippage, fracture, absorption, or subsidence of graft have been noted. Thus, in such a scenario, posterior stabilization is required to prevent complications.[15,16] The anterior procedure has limitations due to associated lung scarring secondary to old or active pulmonary tuberculosis, as well as such potential disadvantages as cage migration, major vessel injury, displacement of the screws, and injury to the viscera. Concomitant osteoporosis associated with infection renders the vertebrae structurally weak, and multiple segment fixation is technically difficult.

The current indication for anterior procedure is pauci-level disease with kyphosis of less than 30 to 40 degrees, which often entails less deformity and less instability. However, in TB of the subaxial cervical spine, the anterior approach remains the standard of care (**Fig. 10.1**).

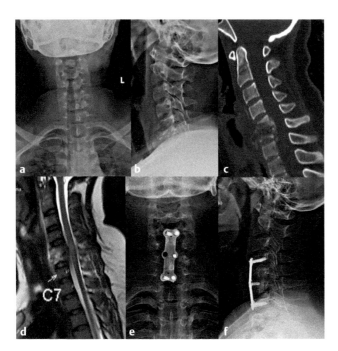

Fig. 10.1 A 27-year-old woman presents with C5-C6 tuberculous spondylodiskitis. **(a,b)** Preoperative radiographs, **(c)** computed tomography (CT), and **(d)** magnetic resonance imaging (MRI) show involvement of the C5 and C6 vertebrae with complete destruction of the vertebral bodies. **(e,f)** Postoperative radiograph after anterior debridement, C4–C7 fusion with an iliac crest graft, and anterior plating.

Combined Approach

A combined anterior and posterior procedure (anterior debridement, grafting, and posterior instrumentation) has an advantage of direct and complete cord decompression and rigid three-column stabilization (**Fig. 10.2**). The addition of posterior instrumentation to augment the anterior interbody fusion has several advantages. It provides rigid fixation in the uninvolved posterior part of the vertebrae, prevents graft-related complications, corrects and prevents the progression of kyphosis, promotes early fusion, and facilitates early mobilization. One-stage surgery is advantageous over two stages as it entails fewer complications, shorter hospital stays, shorter operative time, and less blood loss. The fusion rate after a circumferential fusion has been reported to be nearly 100%.[17]

In active disease, the posterior procedure followed by an anterior procedure facilitates restoring sagittal alignment, placing an adequately sized graft or cage, and producing compressive forces on the anterior graft. However, the selection of the first approach depends on the surgeon's preference. Moon et al[18] described a two-stage procedure in which posterior instrumentation was performed first, followed by anterior decompression and bone grafting 2 to 3 weeks later. Sundararaj et al[19] performed a single-stage combined approach through two separate incisions with equivalent results. Single-stage procedure using a single incision (T-shaped incision) was described by Jain et al[20] for anterior debridement, strut graft, and posterior instrumentation. However, the need to perform two surgeries on a physiologically compromised patient is a major deterrent to using the combined approach in many patients. Indications for the combined approach would be multisegment contiguous TB (especially in the thoracolumbar junction), revision surgery, and significant kyphosis. Recent advances use principles of minimally invasive surgery to reduce the morbidity of combined procedures.

Posterior Procedure

The posterior approach, being more familiar and associated with minimal complications, is now being adapted worldwide for surgical management of thoracic and lumbar spinal TB. The advantages of the posterior approach include familiarity, the ability to achieve circumferential decompression, stronger three-column fixation with pedicle screws, safe performance of anterior debridement by extended approaches, and avoiding entry into the thoracic and abdominal cavity. In the active stage of the disease, when the deformity is mobile, decompression and stabilization of the spine using pedicle screw instrumentation through a posterior-only approach is feasible.

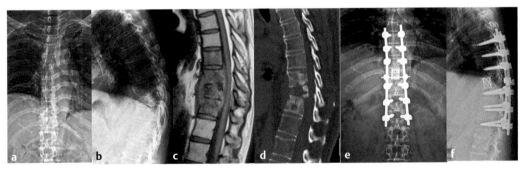

Fig. 10.2 A 49-year-old man presents with multilevel tuberculosis (T8– T11) spondylodiskitis with T10 pathological collapse. **(a,b)** Preoperative radiographs, **(c)** MRI, and **(d)** CT. **(e,f)** Postoperative radiographs after global reconstruction using the combined anteroposterior procedure, showing anterior reconstruction of the defect after debridement with a cylindrical cage and posterior pedicle screw fixation.

In patients with significant anterior column destruction in the thoracic and lumbar region, anterior column reconstruction is performed either through costotransversectomy or through the transpedicular or transforaminal route followed by pedicle screw instrumentation.

Posterior Instrumentation with or without Decompression

Posterior instrumentation alone for the flexible tuberculous kyphosis realigns the spine, maintains the stability, arrests the kyphosis, and hastens healing. Posterior instrumentation with or without decompression is also indicated in cases with pauci-level disease and junctional tuberculosis. Because the TB spine heals by spontaneous bony fusion, anterior debridement may not be necessary in patients with minimal vertebral destruction in the presence of a stable environment. Güven et al[21] reported a 98% cure rate with posterior spinal fusion without any debridement in 87 patients with 10 years of follow-up. Laminectomy alone is indicated only in posterior column TB with neurologic deficit due to either abscess or granulation tissue. In children with spine-at-risk signs, posterior-only stabilization can be done to prevent instability and progression of kyphosis. Posterior instrumentation also helps in the correction of the kyphosis through the growth arrest of the posterior column when it is performed before the age of 10 or 11 years.[13]

Global Reconstruction Through an All-Posterior Approach

With the advent of newer surgical techniques and instrumentations, the approach to the disease has evolved from an anterior to a posterior-only technique. In the active stage of the disease and in lesser deformities (< 30 degrees), it is the authors' practice to perform a primary posterior column shortening to achieve correction. No spinal column distraction or lengthening is performed, so as to allow for adequate interbody contact that facilitates good vertebral body healing (**Fig. 10.3**). In patients with significant anterior column destruction, posterior instrumentation corrects the flexible deformity but creates a bony gap in the anterior column. This defect should be reconstructed with strut grafts or titanium cages with grafts through a transpedicular, transfacetal, or costotransversectomy approach (**Fig. 10.4**). Transfacetal and transpedicular approaches are used for pauci-level TB in the thoracic and lumbar spine. The choice between these two approaches is based on the amount of destruction of the superior half of the inferior vertebrae. The costotransversectomy approach is indicated in patients with multisegmental contiguous involvement.

Zhang et al[22] reported excellent results without recurrence or progression of kyphosis. The all-posterior approach has the following advantages: multiple-level fixation, better deformity correction, excellent exposure for cir-

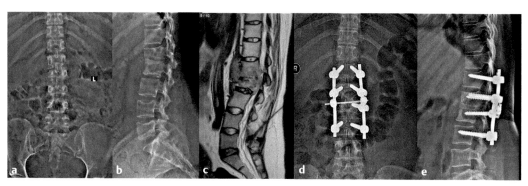

Fig. 10.3 A 28-year-old woman presents with pauci-level (L1-L2) tuberculous spondylodiskitis. **(a,b)** Preoperative radiographs and **(c)** MRI show paradiskal involvement of disease and more destruction of the L2 vertebral body. **(d,e)** Postoperative radiographs after posterior decompression, instrumentation, and compression of the anterior elements without reconstruction.

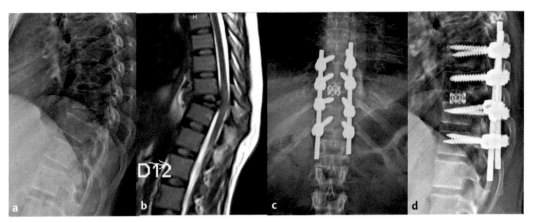

Fig. 10.4 A 30-year-old woman presents with T10 tuberculous spondylodiskitis. **(a)** Preoperative radiograph and **(b)** MRI show T10 vertebra plana. **(c,d)** Postoperative radiographs after global reconstruction through an all-posterior approach: anterior debridement, cage insertion, and posterior pedicle screw fixation.

cumferential spinal cord decompression, and the possibility of anterior reconstruction.

Surgical Technique

After exposing the spine through a posterior approach, pedicle screws are inserted proximally and distally based on the bone quality and the number of the affected vertebrae. In the lumbar spine, it is important to save motion segments, and it is our practice to insert screws into the upper half of the proximal affected vertebrae especially in pauci-level disease. After confirming the position of the screws radiologically, a temporary stabilizing rod is connected on one side. In pauci-level disease, laminectomy/laminotomy and facetectomy are performed. The extension of bony destruction inferior to the level of the pedicle necessitates pedicle removal. Debridement of the anterior lesion is done using straight and curved curettes or shavers, leaving a thin bridge of bone posteriorly that is removed at the end of the debridement. The paravertebral abscess usually drains during this step. If multiple contiguous vertebrae are affected, the anterior part needs to be approached with a one- or two-level costotransversectomy. In the thoracic spine, one or two exiting nerve roots at the level of disease need to be sacrificed for an adequate safe approach. In severe deformity, a similar procedure is performed on the other side. The cavity can then be packed with an appropriately sized tricortical graft or titanium cage packed with graft. It is also vital to pack corticocancellous graft over the circumference of the cage. It is our practice to use a titanium rectangular cage in pauci-segment disease and an oval cylindrical mesh cage in multisegment disease. This is then followed by insertion of the second rod and application of compression to load the anterior column.

Outcomes of Different Approaches

Anterior and posterior instrumentation are equally effective in correcting a deformity and maintaining the correction, as well as in foci clearance, spinal cord decompression, and relieving pain. Moon et al[18] and Chen et al[23] achieved remarkable correction of the kyphotic deformity, with negligible loss of correction, after surgery (1 to 3 degrees) using the anterior approach.[18,23] However, Talu et al,[24] comparing the two groups, noted a postoperative increase in kyphosis of more than 10 degree in 21 of 57 patients who underwent the anterior procedure alone, whereas no such kyphotic progression or graft complications were noted in 70 patients in whom a combined anterior-posterior procedure was done. Similar results demonstrating the superiority of the posterior-only approach in correcting and maintaining the deformity have been reported by others.[25] Liu et al,[26] in a meta-analysis, concluded that the posterior approach has the same clinical efficacy as the anterior approach, but with a shorter operation time, less blood loss, a shorter hospital stay, and fewer complications when compared with the combined posterior and anterior approach. The prognosis regarding neurologic recovery depends on many factors. Neurologic recovery is better in patients with active disease, early presentation, less severe deficit, lesser deformity, and in children. We believe that the most important factor causing neurologic deficit in active disease is the presence of instability, and hence we advise early stabilization with decompression and fusion in all patients with a neurologic deficit. Late presentation, prolonged neurologic deficit, old age, and associated comorbidities do not favor a good neurologic outcome.

Surgery by the anterior, posterior, or combined approach will be successful if the surgical principles are adequately executed. The final decision on the surgical approach should be based on the surgeon's experience and expertise. Strict adherence to the chemotherapy regimen is mandatory in all surgical patients to achieve a good clinical outcome.

Minimally Invasive Surgery in Spinal Tuberculosis

Minimally invasive surgery (MIS) techniques such as video-assisted thoracoscopic debridement, posterolateral endoscopic debridement, transforaminal lumbar interbody fusion (TLIF), and extreme lateral interbody fusion (XLIF) are now being used frequently with successful results. Good success has been reported with these techniques when they are used either as a stand-alone procedure or in combination with open procedures. They are discussed in Chapter 13.

Posttubercular Kyphotic Deformity

Although the risk of significant progression of deformity is very low in adults, in children the kyphotic deformity continues to progress even after disease healing. Severe kyphotic deformities are usually the result of childhood spinal TB and can be identified by spine-at-risk radiological signs in the active stage.[14] Children can also develop buckling collapse, leading to progressive kyphosis of more than 120 degrees.[27] Hence, it is essential that the prevention of deformity be an integral part of any treatment schedule in spinal TB. The clinical presentation varies depending on the severity of the deformity and includes back pain, costopelvic impingement, secondary cardiorespiratory problems, postural problems, and late-onset neurologic deficits. A neurologic deficit can develop due to prolonged stretching of the spinal cord over the kyphos, resulting in cord atrophy and myelomalacia, and is known as late-onset Pott's paraplegia in healed disease.[4] Dynamic factors due to nonunion and instability are other contributing factors. Compensatory hyperlordosis at adjacent levels may lead to accelerated facet degeneration and ligamentum flavum hypertrophy causing neurologic deficit. Rarely, a neurologic deficit can occur due to reactivation of the disease.

Surgery in Late-Onset Kyphosis

Correction of an established kyphosis is a herculean and hazardous task, with a high rate of complications. The management of late-onset kyphosis depends on its severity, the presence of a neurologic deficit, the general condition of the patient, and, most importantly, the experience of the surgeon. A kyphosis of 30 to 70 degrees is usually due to pauci-level disease and can be managed by either an anteroposterior approach or a pedicle substraction osteotomy. Bezer et al[28] reported on a 5-year follow-up study of 16 patients with tuberculous kyphosis who underwent pedicle subtraction osteotomy. The mean preoperative kyphosis of 30 degrees was corrected to 12 degrees. Forward sagittal balance was reduced from 68 mm to 12 mm. All patients achieved fusion, and none had neurologic complications. Similarly, others have observed excellent deformity correction (kyphosis reduction to under 50% of the preoperative magnitude and high fusion rates with pedicle subtraction osteotomy).[29]

Chunguang et al[30] reported on 16 children with kyphotic deformity of the spine in healed stages of TB who underwent anterior release, decompression, deformity correction, and instrumented fusion, followed by posterior osteotomy, deformity correction, and pedicle screw instrumented fusion. The mean preoperative angle of kyphosis was 55.8 degrees that reduced to 21.7 degrees postoperatively.

Posterior vertebral column resection (PVCR) is indicated in deformities greater than 60 degrees (**Fig. 10.5**). There are challenges in performing a PVCR in posttuberculous kyphosis, as opposed to in congenital or other severe kyphosis, because multiple vertebral bodies are involved in the postinfectious fusion mass, the anatomic landmarks are distorted, and adhesions frequently tether the thecal sac to the anterior structures of the spinal column. The insertion of an anterior cage and compression from behind (closing-opening maneuver) in the PVCR osteotomy avoids undue stretching or kinking of the spinal cord.[31] Specific attention should be paid to avoiding overzealous correction and shortening of the cord, and to preventing hypotension. Rajasekaran[32] reported on 17 patients with severe late TB kyphosis (10 thoracolumbar, six thoracic, and one lumbar) treated with a one-stage closing-opening PVCR. The number of periapical vertebrae involved ranged from two to five. The preoperative kyphosis averaged 69.8 degrees and the postoperative kyphosis averaged 32.8 degrees, with a mean kyphosis correction of 57%. No patient with normal preoperative neurologic status showed deterioration.[32]

In patients with buckling collapse and severe deformities, the aim is to prevent development of a neurologic deficit or to salvage slowly progressive neurology. However, a kyphosis of greater than 120 degrees is difficult to treat

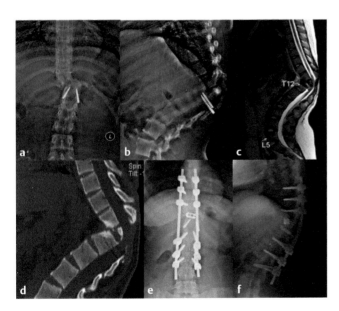

Fig. 10.5 A 18-year-old woman presents with posttubercular kyphosis. She underwent surgery in childhood, followed by implant removal. **(a,b)** Preoperative radiographs show translation in the anteroposterior plane and significant kyphosis. **(c)** MRI shows stretching of the cord over the T11 internal gibbus. **(d)** CT shows a posterior laminar defect. **(e,f)** Postoperative radiographs after closing-opening wedge osteotomy (COWO) with good correction in both planes.

even with PCVR. Wong et al[33] reported on a series of patients treated with decompression of the internal gibbus and stabilization of kyphosis, with strut bone grafting via the costotransversectomy approach; 40% of patients had neurologic improvement and none had neurologic deterioration after the surgery. The management of post-TB kyphosis carries a significant risk of neurologic injury and blood loss, and should be performed by experienced surgeons at specialized centers.

Chapter Summary

The objectives of treatment of spinal tuberculosis are to control infection, prevent neural damage, and prevent and correct deformities. The effective healing through conservative management has been time and again demonstrable and remains the mainstay of treatment. Surgical intervention is warranted in tuberculosis of the spine that is complicated by neural deficit and deformity. With better understanding of biomechanics and the natural history of spinal TB, prevention of deformity in the active stage of the disease has become one of the main strategies. The principles of surgery in spinal TB include debridement, decompression of the spinal canal, correction of deformity, reconstruction of the anterior defect, and instrumentation. Currently, more emphasis is being placed on restoring the sagittal balance. The choice of approach is made based on the needs of patient, the level of the lesion, the amount of vertebral body loss, and, most importantly, on the experience and preference of the surgeon. The anterior approach is rewarding and most commonly used in the subaxial cervical spine. The morbidity associated with the anterior approach in the thoracolumbar spine precludes its use, in spite of the ease with which the anterior structures can be debrided and decompressed effectively. In thoracic and lumbar TB, the posterior approach is currently preferred, as anterior reconstruction is still possible in addi-

tion to the versatile pedicle screw instrumentation now available. Fluoroscopy- or CT-guided minimally invasive biopsy enables better targeting and aids in retrieving adequate samples from accurate areas. MIS has also gained popularity recently. Irrespective of the approach used, the success of the procedure depends on following the surgical principles and on strict adherence to antituberculous chemotherapy.

Pearls

- Spinal instrumentation helps to enhance stability, minimize graft dislodgement, correct deformity, and facilitate early mobilization and rehabilitation of patients.
- During debridement of the spinal infection in the vertebral body, an extensive debridement to the extent of the bleeding bone surfaces is not mandatory. Adequate debridement to remove the infective focus, relieving the spinal cord compression, and providing stability are the goals of surgical intervention.
- Children with spine-at-risk signs need posterior spinal fusion to avoid the development of late-onset kyphosis.
- Elderly patients with spinal tuberculosis need a thorough workup for surgical intervention, as they are prone to perioperative complications.
- In cervical tuberculosis, the anterior approach is the preferred method that enables safe debridement, decompression, and spinal fixation.

Pitfalls

- When using an all-posterior approach, short segment fixation should be avoided and a minimum of two spinal segments need to be fixed adjacent to the lesion.
- When the anterior vertebral defect is wide, anterior reconstruction using a cage or a strut graft is essential to avoid implant failure.
- The use of titanium implants is strongly advised in the presence of spinal tubercular infections, as debridement and grafting alone does not suffice and entails complications. The use of implants has been found to be safe, with less risk of implant biofilm in tuberculosis.
- Tuberculosis is predominantly a medical disease, and, even with a good surgical treatment, chemotherapy still holds the key for successful patient outcomes.

References
Five Must-Read References

1. Tuli SM. Historical aspects of Pott's disease (spinal tuberculosis) management. Eur Spine J 2013;22(4, Suppl 4):529–538
2. Hodgson AR, Stock FE. Anterior spinal fusion a preliminary communication on the radical treatment of Pott's disease and Pott's paraplegia. Br J Surg 1956; 44:266–275
3. Medical Research Council Working Party on Tuberculosis of the Spine. A 15-year assessment of controlled trials of the management of tuberculosis of the spine in Korea and Hong Kong. Thirteenth Report of the Medical Research Council Working Party on Tuberculosis of the Spine. J Bone Joint Surg Br 1998; 80:456–462
4. Cheung WY, Luk KD. Clinical and radiological outcomes after conservative treatment of TB spondylitis: is the 15 years' follow-up in the MRC study long enough? Eur Spine J 2013;22(4, Suppl 4):594–602
5. Oga M, Arizono T, Takasita M, Sugioka Y. Evaluation of the risk of instrumentation as a foreign body in spinal tuberculosis. Clinical and biologic study. Spine 1993;18:1890–1894
6. Rajasekaran S, Kanna RM, Shetty AP. Pathophysiology and treatment of spinal tuberculosis. JBJS Rev 2014;2:e4
7. Ge Z, Wang Z, Wei M. Measurement of the concentration of three antituberculosis drugs in the focus of spinal tuberculosis. Eur Spine J 2008;17:1482–1487
8. Shetty A, Kanna RM, Rajasekaran S. TB spine—current aspects on clinical presentation, diagnosis, and management options. Semin Spine Surg 2016;28:150–162
9. Rajasekaran S. The problem of deformity in spinal tuberculosis. Clin Orthop Relat Res 2002;398:85–92
10. Lee SH, Sung JK, Park YM. Single-stage transpedicular decompression and posterior instrumentation in treatment of thoracic and thoracolumbar spinal tuberculosis: a retrospective case series. J Spinal Disord Tech 2006;19:595–602
11. Broner FA, Garland DE, Zigler JE. Spinal infections in the immunocompromised host. Orthop Clin North Am 1996;27:37–46
12. Jain AK, Kumar J. Tuberculosis of spine: neurological deficit. Eur Spine J 2013;22(4, Suppl 4):624–633
13. Rajasekaran S. The natural history of post-tubercular kyphosis in children. Radiological signs which predict late increase in deformity. J Bone Joint Surg Br 2001;83:954–962
14. Rajasekaran S, Shanmugasundaram TK. Prediction of the angle of gibbus deformity in tuberculosis of the spine. J Bone Joint Surg Am 1987;69:503–509
15. Rajasekaran S, Soundarapandian S. Progression of kyphosis in tuberculosis of the spine treated by anterior arthrodesis. J Bone Joint Surg Am 1989;71:1314–1323
16. Benli IT, Alanay A, Akalin S, et al. Comparison of anterior instrumentation systems and the results of minimum 5 years follow-up in the treatment of tuberculosis spondylitis. Kobe J Med Sci 2004;50:167–180
17. Wang B, Ozawa H, Tanaka Y, Matsumoto F, Aizawa T, Kokubun S. One-stage lateral rhachotomy and posterior spinal fusion with compression hooks for Pott's paralysis in the elderly. J Orthop Surg (Hong Kong) 2006;14:310–314
18. Moon MS, Woo YK, Lee KS, Ha KY, Kim SS, Sun DH. Posterior instrumentation and anterior interbody fusion for tuberculous kyphosis of dorsal and lumbar spines. Spine 1995;20:1910–1916
19. Sundararaj GD, Behera S, Ravi V, Venkatesh K, Cherian VM, Lee V. Role of posterior stabilisation in the management of tuberculosis of the dorsal and lumbar spine. J Bone Joint Surg Br 2003;85:100–106
20. Jain AK, Dhammi IK, Jain S, Kumar J. Simultaneously anterior decompression and posterior instrumentation by extrapleural retroperitoneal approach in thoracolumbar lesions. Indian J Orthop 2010;44: 409–416
21. Güven O, Kumano K, Yalçin S, Karahan M, Tsuji S. A single stage posterior approach and rigid fixation for preventing kyphosis in the treatment of spinal tuberculosis. Spine 1994;19:1039–1043
22. Zhang HQ, Li JS, Zhao SS, et al. Surgical management for thoracic spinal tuberculosis in the elderly: posterior only versus combined posterior and anterior approaches. Arch Orthop Trauma Surg 2012;132: 1717–1723
23. Chen WJ, Wu CC, Jung CH, Chen LH, Niu CC, Lai PL. Combined anterior and posterior surgeries in the treatment of spinal tuberculous spondylitis. Clin Orthop Relat Res 2002;398:50–59
24. Talu U, Gogus A, Ozturk C, Hamzaoglu A, Domanic U. The role of posterior instrumentation and fusion after anterior radical debridement and fusion in the surgical treatment of spinal tuberculosis: experience of 127 cases. J Spinal Disord Tech 2006;19:554–559
25. Garg B, Kandwal P, Nagaraja UB, Goswami A, Jayaswal A. Anterior versus posterior procedure for surgical treatment of thoracolumbar tuberculosis: A retrospective analysis. Indian J Orthop 2012;46: 165–170
26. Liu J, Wan L, Long X, Huang S, Dai M, Liu Z. Efficacy and safety of posterior versus combined posterior and anterior approach for the treatment of spinal tuberculosis: a meta-analysis. World Neurosurg 2015; 83:1157–1165

27. Rajasekaran S. Buckling collapse of the spine in childhood spinal tuberculosis. Clin Orthop Relat Res 2007; 460:86–92

28. Bezer M, Kucukdurmaz F, Guven O. Transpedicular decancellation osteotomy in the treatment of post-tuberculous kyphosis. J Spinal Disord Tech 2007;20: 209–215

29. Kalra KP, Dhar SB, Shetty G, Dhariwal Q. Pedicle subtraction osteotomy for rigid post-tuberculous kyphosis. J Bone Joint Surg Br 2006;88:925–927

30. Chunguang Z, Limin L, Rigao C, et al. Surgical treatment of kyphosis in children in healed stages of spinal tuberculosis. J Pediatr Orthop 2010;30:271–276

31. Boachie-Adjei O, Papadopoulos EC, Pellisé F, et al. Late treatment of tuberculosis-associated kyphosis: literature review and experience from a SRS-GOP site. Eur Spine J 2013;22(4, Suppl 4):641–646

32. Rajasekaran S. Kyphotic deformity in spinal tuberculosis and its management. Int Orthop 2012;36:359–365

33. Wong YW, Leong JCY, Luk KD. Direct internal kyphectomy for severe angular tuberculous kyphosis. Clin Orthop Relat Res 2007;460:124–129

11

Pediatric Spinal Infections

S. Rajasekaran, Rishi M. Kanna, and Ajoy Prasad Shetty

Introduction

Infections of the spine are rare in children, and can be classified as acute and chronic infections based on the clinical presentation. Acute infections are caused by pyogenic organisms, commonly by *Staphylococcus* or *Streptococcus* species or by gram-negative organisms. Chronic infections are granulomatous in nature and are most commonly caused by tubercular bacilli and rarely by fungus and parasites. Pyogenic diskitis is the most commonly encountered form of vertebral infection in developed nations, whereas tuberculosis is more common in developing countries. Infection usually develops from hematogenous spread of bacteria, and uncommonly by direct inoculation, contiguous spread from adjacent structures, or iatrogenic causes. Due to the intact vascularity of the disk in children, the primary focus of infection in the spine is the intervertebral disk; infection then spreads into the epidural space and vertebral body. Diagnosis is difficult because of vague clinical symptoms, the child's inability to communicate, the lack of standard diagnostic tests, and a delay in seeking specialist medical care. Early diagnosis and management is important, as good results can be obtained even with conservative treatment in the initial stages. A delay in diagnosis can lead to sepsis, neurologic deficits, spinal deformity, or even death in children with pyogenic spondylitis. In chronic infections, kyphosis and neu-

rologic deficit are the important sequelae in neglected infections. Management is predominantly medical in both acute and chronic spinal infections and involves identification of the organism, appropriate antimicrobial chemotherapy, and supportive treatment. Surgical treatment is rarely indicated in patients with extensive vertebral destruction, abscess formation, neurologic deficits, deformity, and severe pain due to instability. Prognosis depends on the rapidity of diagnosis, the type of organism, the severity of vertebral damage, and the immune status and general condition of the patient.

Acute Pyogenic Spinal Infections

The current incidence of pyogenic vertebral infection has been observed to be 1 per 250,000 in the general population, accounting for approximately 2 to 4% of all osteomyelitis.[1] The exact incidence of pediatric pyogenic spinal infections is not clear because of the rarity of its occurrence. The age at diagnosis of pyogenic diskitis in children is generally 2 to 8 years. Although any level of the spine can be affected, the incidence is more common in the lumbar region (> 50% of cases).[2] Because of its rarity and vague initial signs and symptoms, diagnosis is often delayed, and the average time to diagnosis is 8 to 10 days after the onset of symptoms. A high index of suspicion is essential to avoid diagnostic delays because the evolving abscess can result in severe compression of the neural structures, and systemic spread of the infection can lead to septicemia, resulting in significant morbidity and mortality.

Etiopathogenesis

Gram-positive cocci (*Staphylococcus aureus* and *Streptococcus pyogenes*) are by far the most common organisms to cause vertebral infection, although other infective organisms, including *Escherichia coli, Pseudomonas, Klebsiella,* and *Proteus,* have also been isolated.[3] In children with sickle cell anemia, *Salmonella* infection is common. Most infections occur due to bacterial spread from a distant site (dermal, respiratory tract, and genitourinary tract) to the spinal column through the bloodstream (hematogenous spread). Several risk factors such as immune deficiency states, long-term systemic administration of steroids, juvenile diabetes mellitus, organ transplantation, malnutrition, chemotherapy for malignancy, infective endocarditis, renal failure, and sickle cell disease have been identified for the development of vertebral infections.

Although the arterial route is the common route of bacterial spread to a vertebra, retrograde seeding of venous blood via Batson's venous plexus and rarely contiguous spread of infection from a nearby infected focus to the vertebra and disk can also produce infective spondylitis. The intervertebral disks in children are vascular until 8 years of age. Hence, unlike adult vertebral infections, primary disk infection is more common in children. In older children, the infection also spreads easily from the subchondral region of the vertebral body due to the abundant blood supply of the trabecular cancellous bone and its rich, cellular marrow. As the blood flow stagnates in the metaphyseal arterial loops just beneath the vertebral end plates, the circulating bacteria readily colonize there, subsequently invading the disk. In pyogenic spondylitis, the involvement is usually focal, but multiple site involvement can occur in immune-compromised patients. As vertebral and diskal destruction proceeds, the vertebral canal can be involved by pus and granulation tissue, which can cause cord compression resulting in a rapid-onset neurologic deficit. Other sequelae include meningitis, sepsis, and rarely death. Severe vertebral deformity and excess abscess formation are uncommon in pyogenic spondylitis.

Clinical Symptoms and Signs

Toddlers and infants with pyogenic spondylitis have a varied clinical presentation, including difficulty in walking, abdominal pain, hip and thigh pain, and refusal to eat. General features of infection, such as fever, malaise, and fatigability, are also present. A high degree of clinical suspicion and a meticulous clinical examination to note the presence of spinal guarding and local spinal tenderness can help in making the diagnosis. In older children, the usual presentation is one of insidious onset back pain and fever. The pain is initially localized to the level of the infection, but vague distribution to the paraspinal areas is also common. Because young children may not directly complain of back pain, a "coin test or quarter test" has been described in which the child is unable to pick up a coin from the floor due to painful restriction of spinal movements.

Neurologic involvement can occur early when compared with tubercular infection, even in the presence of minimal vertebral body collapse and thin epidural abscess. If neurologic involvement is suspected, a meticulous neurologic examination, including per-rectal examination to detect early cauda equina compression, is essential. Ideally the neurologic examination should be repeated and documented at regular intervals as the child will be unable to complain about sudden neurologic worsening.

Investigations

Blood tests to evaluate the presence of infection including total cell count, differential cell count, erythrocyte sedimentation rate (ESR), and C-reactive protein (CRP) are performed. These investigations provide only a glimpse of the diagnosis and are neither specific nor sensitive for pyogenic spondylitis. Leukocytosis (> 15,000 cells/mm^3) is present in < 50% in patients with pyogenic spondylitis. Elevated ESR and CRP levels are the most common laboratory abnormality and are excellent indicators of acute inflammation but remain nonspecific in the diagnosis of infective spondylitis. Both are more helpful in assessing the response to treatment. Decreasing values would indicate a good response to antibiotic treatment.

Urine and blood cultures are performed in all patients, but are positive in only 40 to 50% of patients with spinal infections. Blood cultures should always be obtained during a febrile episode and prior to administration of antibiotics. Positive results are of immense value in choosing the appropriate antibiotic treatment. If all cultures turn out to be negative, then biopsy is required to isolate tissue specimen for culture.

Radiological Studies

Plain radiographs are notoriously normal in the first 2 to 3 weeks after infection. Loss of delineation of subchondral bone, vertebral lucencies, and destruction of the end plates with narrowing of the disk space are the earliest changes but are usually seen by the end of 3 weeks. In advanced disease, destruction of vertebral bodies, collapse with kyphosis and features of spinal instability may be evident. Magnetic resonance imaging (MRI) is the investigation of choice due to its ability to depict changes even in the early stages of the disease (**Fig. 11.1**). Hence, MRI should be performed with a low threshold to diagnose infection in the early stages. MRI has a high sensitivity of 96%, a specificity of 92%, and an accuracy of 94% in patients with disk space infections.[4] T1-weighted images show decreased signal intensity changes in the vertebral bodies and disk spaces. T2-weighted images show increased signal intensity in the vertebral disk and body. Short tau inversion recovery (STIR) sequences and contrast images are also highly useful in diagnosing infection in the early stages. It also clearly documents the location and size of epidural abscess, the presence of sequestrum within the canal, the extent of compromise of the spinal canal, the degree of compression of the spinal cord, and any signal intensity changes in the cord.

Computed tomography (CT) is performed in select situations and is considered to be more sensitive in assessing the degree of bone destruction and in examining the surrounding soft tissues. It is also used as a guide for accurate placement of the Jamshidi needle while performing a percutaneous biopsy. A radionuclear

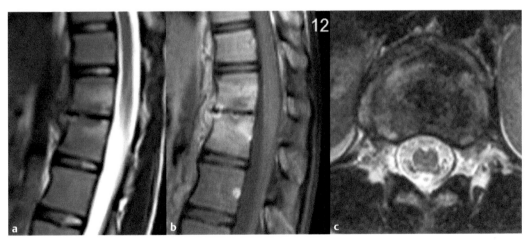

Fig. 11.1 Magnetic resonance imaging (MRI) is effective in diagnosing early spinal infections. The typical features of early spondylodiskitis include bright signal on **(a)** T2-weighted images and low signal on **(b)** T1-weighted images in the affected vertebral bodies, associated with end-plate disruption. **(c)** Axial T2 images show a thin rim of paravertebral abscess.

bone scan with technetium-99m is a sensitive test (> 90%) for the early diagnosis of pyogenic vertebral osteomyelitis. Although expensive, a radioactive gallium scan is more specific, with 80 to 85% specificity rates. Gallium localizes inflammatory lesions well and, when combined with technetium, demonstrates virtually all pyogenic vertebral infections. But the lesions are not well localized by radionuclide scans, and the scans do not demonstrate the true extent of infection. Thus, MRI has superseded radionuclide scans and remains the gold standard imaging test.

Histopathology

Computed tomography guided or fluoroscopy enabled percutaneous biopsy of the infected vertebra or disk is advised where a tissue biopsy is required. Although cultures are positive in only 50 to 60% of patients with an infection, histological findings are invariably confirmative. Trocar biopsies are better than fine-needle aspiration because a larger amount of material from the infected area can be obtained. If blood cultures and percutaneous biopsy techniques fail to identify the infecting organism, open surgical debridement and biopsy should be performed. An open surgical biopsy has the highest success rate for positive culture findings (up to 90%) and helps in diagnostic confirmation.[5]

Management

Conservative treatment is usually successful in most children, especially in the early stages of the disease. Conservative treatment involves a combination of rest, immobilization with a brace or cast, and antibiotic therapy. The success rate with conservative treatment is high when the diagnosis is certain, the infective organism is known, and appropriate antibiotics can be instituted before the development of severe destruction or neurologic complications. Before culture results are received, it is prudent to start empirical antibiotic therapy with a third-generation cephalosporin and oxacillin/clindamycin. There is no clear consensus on the exact duration of antibiotic therapy, but generally intravenous antibiotics, initiated based on culture and sensitivity patterns, are given for a period of 3 to 4 weeks followed by an equal period of oral antibiotic therapy. Serial monitoring with ESR and CRP levels is useful to evaluate the response to antibiotics. Failure of resolution of clinical symptoms, a persistently high ESR, and progressive destruction in radiographs would indicate the failure of conservative therapy.

Surgical Treatment

Surgical treatment is required in the few patients whose symptoms persist despite antibiotic care, as well as in patients with sepsis, in patients in whom the organism could not be isolated, and in patients with an ambiguous diagnosis, a neurologic deficit, or increasing kyphosis. Surgery should aim to obtain adequate material for both bacteriological and histological diagnosis, to adequately decompress the neural structures, and to provide stability with reconstruction of the spinal column. The safety of titanium implants in the presence of spinal infection is now well documented (**Fig. 11.2**). They allow little biofilm formation and lack bioadhesive properties, which prevents the adhesion of bacteria to the implants. In children with epidural abscess without significant vertebral destruction, laminectomy for drainage of the abscess can be performed.

Chronic Pediatric Spinal Infections

Chronic infections of the spine in children are usually caused by tuberculous bacilli and rarely by fungi and parasites. These infections are common in developing countries due to poor hygiene, crowded conditions, decreased access to health care, and the lack of knowledge about spinal infections. In developed countries, these infections are rare, and children with immunosuppression and immigrant population are more commonly afflicted than the general population.

It is important to recognize that childhood spinal tuberculosis differs from adult infection

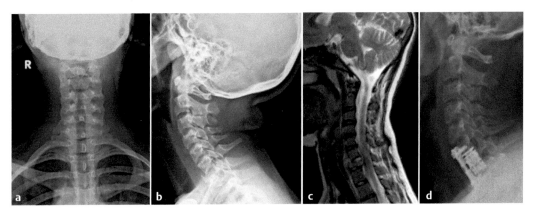

Fig. 11.2 A 16-year-old child presents with severe axial neck pain of 3 months' duration. Although the anteroposterior (AP) radiograph **(a)** is unremarkable, the lateral radiograph **(b)** and the sagittal T2 MRI **(c)** show C7 vertebral body destruction. **(d)** The patient underwent anterior corpectomy and stabilization from C6 to T1.

in both its severity and its clinical behavior. The pediatric vertebral bodies are very vulnerable for rapid and complete destruction during the acute phase, and thus frequently develop major defects of the anterior vertebral column. The pediatric spine is also more flexible, making it susceptible to greater deformity and instability than the adult spine during the active phase of the disease. Although the deformity does not change after healing and consolidation in adults, children continue to exhibit progressive deformity, for better or worse, until growth is complete. As a result, children with spinal tuberculosis require a careful follow-up until they are grown.

Microbiology and Pathophysiology

Tuberculosis is caused by a bacillus of the *Mycobacterium tuberculosis* complex. Akin to pyogenic infections, vertebral infection by the bacillus results from hematogenous dissemination from a primary focus elsewhere in the system, commonly the lungs, lymph nodes, or kidneys. Spread of the organism can also occur through the lymphatics from the viscera to the adjacent vertebral segments; for example, pulmonary tuberculosis can spread to the thoracic spine.

Following infection in the vertebral marrow, the chronic inflammatory response is characterized by slow accumulation of macrophages and monocytes. The tubercle bacilli are phagocytosed, and their lipid is dispersed throughout the cytoplasm of macrophages, transforming the macrophages into epithelioid cells, which are characteristic of the tuberculous reaction. Another characteristic feature of tuberculous lesion is the presence of Langhans giant cells, which are formed by the coalescence of a number of epithelioid cells. With progressive destruction, caseation necrosis occurs and adjacent lesions coalesce to form a large abscess, and because it is a chronic infection, the acute features of inflammation such as warmth and redness are absent (cold abscess).

The most common pattern of tubercular spinal infection in adults is the paradiskal type, in which the bacilli lodge in the subchondral marrow on either side of the disk. In children, the disk retains its blood supply until approximately 8 years of age, and so the bacilli affect and destroy the vertebral body and disk simultaneously (centrum or complete type of pattern). Due to the weaker immune response of the child and the cartilaginous nature of the vertebral body, extensive vertebral destruction and exuberant abscess formation are more common in children. The other types of spinal tuberculosis are the anterior type (abscess formation beneath the anterior longitudinal ligament), the posterior type (isolated involvement of the posterior elements), and the nonosseous type (extensive abscess formation with very little bony destruction).

Clinical Presentation

Unlike pyogenic spondylitis, tuberculous lesions have a much more insidious onset, and the clinical symptoms often develop over a period of 1 to 2 months. Back pain localized to the affected site and aggravated with spinal movements is the usual presenting feature. The affected child may need to support his trunk by placing the hands on the couch while sitting or holding the neck by the hands when the cervical spine is affected (**Fig. 11.3**). Constitutional symptoms of malaise, loss of appetite and weight, evening rise of temperature, and night sweats are also observed in up to 60% of patients.[6] A paravertebral cold abscess is a diagnostic feature of spinal tuberculosis. It may be clinically evident, either in the paraspinal area or the abscess may tract distally along the fascial planes to present remotely away from the vertebral lesion (**Fig. 11.4**).

Neurologic compromise occurs in 30 to 75% of the patients with spinal tuberculosis.[7] Although children have more severe destruction, they have a lesser incidence of neurologic involvement, probably due to the relative larger canal diameter and more flexibility of the spine. Children can present with neurologic involvement both in the active and healed phase of the disease. In active lesions, it is the result of direct compression of the spinal cord by an abscess or inflammatory granulation tissue; in the healed stages, neurologic deficit occurs after many years due to gradual stretching of the cord over a bony ridge at the apex of the kyphosis.

Kyphosis is an important sequelae of spinal tuberculosis. Classically, tuberculosis affects and destroys the anterior structures of the vertebral column in more than 90% of patients. As disease progresses, the vertebral body collapses, resulting in kyphosis (**Fig. 11.5**). The severity of acute kyphosis that develops during the active phase of the disease is mainly influenced by the severity of vertebral destruction, the level of the lesion, and the age of the patient. Children with complete involvement of one vertebral body, multiple adjacent vertebral involvement, thoracic lesions, and those less than 10 years of age have significant kyphosis during the active stages of the disease. The kyphotic collapse is less extensive in lumbar lesions due to lumbar lordosis, the large size of the intervertebral disks, and the sagittal orientation of the facet joints. Children younger than 10 years of age have been observed to have greater deformity due to their soft vertebral bodies and their weaker posterior stabilizing structures.

In a long-term follow-up of 15 years in 63 children afflicted with spinal tuberculosis,

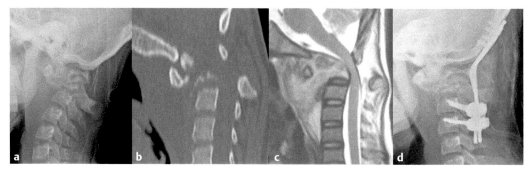

Fig. 11.3 A 13-year-old child presented with cervical pain of 3 months duration with subtle myelopathy. The lateral radiograph **(a)**, sagittal CT **(b)** shows the complete destruction of C1 and C2 vertebra with atlantoaxial instability and dislocation suggestive of upper cervical tuberculosis. The sagittal MR image shows extensive prevertebral abscess formation and cord compression at the level of C1 **(c)**. The patient has been treated by posterior decompression, abscess drainage, and fusion from occiput to C4 **(d)**.

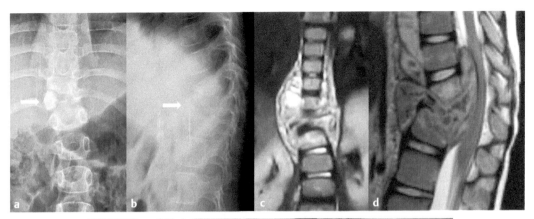

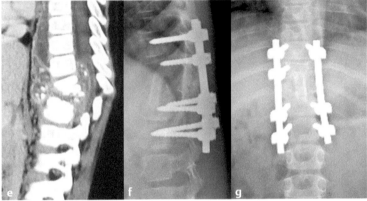

Fig. 11.4 A 9-year-old child presents with T12-L1 tuberculosis, paraplegia, and extensive cold abscess. **(a,b)** The radiographs show vertebral collapse and local kyphosis. **(c–e)** MRI scans show extensive abscess formation in the perivertebral space, epidural abscess, cord compression, and multiple vertebral destruction. **(f)** The sagittal CT shows the extent of bony destruction. **(g)** The patient is treated with modified Hong Kong surgery through anterior debridement and reconstruction with an autofibular graft and supplemental posterior stabilization.

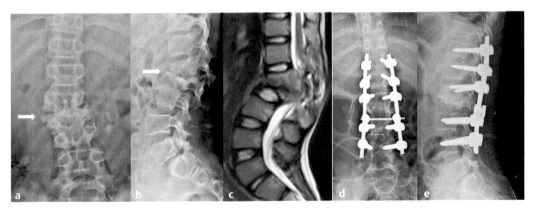

Fig. 11.5 Acute kyphosis in a 13-year-old boy with L1-2 tuberculosis. The AP and lateral radiographs show the vertebral damage and local kyphosis about 30 degrees **(a,b)**. Sagittal MR images show abscess formation and vertebral collapse causing cord compression **(c)**. He has been treated by posterior decompression, transpedicular abscess drainage, posterior column shortening with Ponte's osteotomy and stabilisation from T11 to L3 **(d,e)**.

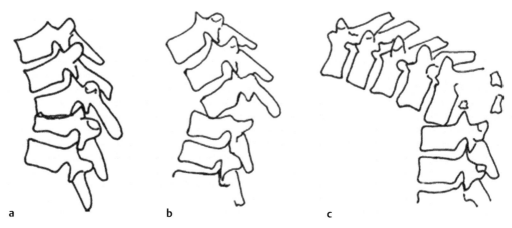

Fig. 11.6 Following destruction of the anterior column, restabilization and healing occurs by one of the three methods. **(a)** In patients with minimally destroyed vertebrae with intact facet joints, restabilization occurs with wide contact area. **(b)** In patients with dislocation of single facet joint, restabilization occurred by point contact. **(c)** In patients with loss of two or three vertebrae, the facets dislocate at multiple levels, and the superior segment rotates by 90 degrees so that its anterior surface can rest on the superior surface of the inferior vertebra.

Rajasekaran et al[8] reported three types of kyphotic collapse with different implications for deformity progression during the period of growth (**Fig. 11.6**). Type A healing was seen in minimal lesions and a paradiskal type of involvement, where the facet joints were intact and there were large areas of contact of vertebral bodies anteriorly. These patients had minimal kyphotic deformity. Type B healing was seen when the vertebral body loss was equivalent to the loss of one vertebral body. When these children were treated nonsurgically, the adjacent vertebrae collapsed and the facet joint at the level of destruction dislocated. The superior vertebra was observed to rotate during the process of descent so that its anteroinferior margin came into point contact with the superior surface of the inferior normal vertebra. This resulted in growth depression at the point of contact. Type C restabilization occurred when the loss increased to more than two vertebral bodies. During the process of disease healing without any surgical intervention, the large anterior column defect necessitated the dislocation of two or more facet joints, and the superior normal vertebra was noted to rotate almost 90 degrees, so that the anterior surface of the superior vertebra comes in contact with the superior surface of the inferior vertebra. This results in an acute angular kyphosis.

Unlike in adults, in whom the deformity is static after cure of the disease, the kyphosis that is residual in children at the completion of chemotherapy is a dynamic deformity with variable progression during growth (**Fig. 11.7**). Three different patterns of progression have been observed depending on the pattern of healing. Type I progression, in which worsening of the deformity occurs during growth, is seen in 39%. Type II progression, in which, after an increase in deformity during the active phase, the deformity shows a progressive and spontaneous correction, is seen is 44%. Type III progression, in which there is no major change during growth, is seen in 17%; these patients have either minimal disease or a lower lumbar lesion.

Four radiological signs that indicate spinal instability have been identified by Rajasekaran[9] to predict the risk of late development of deformity in childhood spinal tuberculosis (**Fig. 11.8**). These signs are easy to identify in radiographs, appear early in the course of the disease, and are useful in identifying children at risk for progression so that surgical stabilization can be suitably advocated. They basically

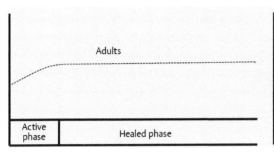

Fig. 11.7 Deformity progression in healed tuberculosis in adults and children. In adults, the deformity remains the same during the healed phase. In children, the deformity can either worsen (type I), remain static (type III), or improve (type II) during the healed phase.

indicate the presence of facet joint dislocation. These four spine-at-risk signs are (1) dislocation of one or more facet joints in the lateral view, (2) retropulsion of the diseased vertebra, (3) lateral translation seen in the anteroposterior view, and (4) the toppling sign. The presence of at least two of these signs during the active phases of treatment of spinal tuberculosis indicates the need for prophylactic surgical stabilization to avoid development of severe kyphosis later.

Diagnostic Tests and Management

The principles of diagnostic testing and the management guidelines are similar to those in adult spinal tuberculosis and are described in detail in Chapters 10 and 11.

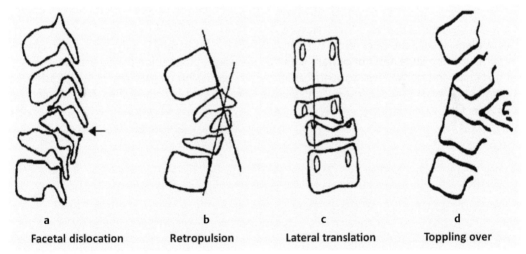

a	b	c	d
Facetal dislocation	**Retropulsion**	**Lateral translation**	**Toppling over**

Fig. 11.8 Rajasekaran's spine-at-risk radiological signs. **(a)** Separation of the facet joint. The facet joint dislocates at the level of the apex of the curve, causing instability and loss of alignment. In severe cases the separation can occur at two levels. **(b)** Posterior retropulsion. This is identified by drawing two lines along the posterior surface of the first upper and lower normal vertebrae. The diseased segments are found to be posterior to the intersection of the lines. **(c)** Lateral translation. This is confirmed when a vertical line drawn through the middle of the pedicle of the first lower normal vertebra does not touch the pedicle of the first upper normal vertebra. **(d)** Toppling sign. In the initial stages of collapse, a line drawn along the anterior surface of the first lower normal vertebra intersects the inferior surface of the first upper normal vertebra. Tilt or toppling occurs when the line intersects higher than the middle of the anterior surface of the first normal upper vertebra.

Chapter Summary

Spinal infection in children can be acute or chronic. Acute infections are caused by pyogenic organisms. Because children are not good at divulging their symptoms, a good clinical history and physical examination are essential to avoid misdiagnosis. Because radiographs can be normal in the crucial first 2 weeks, MRI should be performed early for appropriate diagnosis. All efforts to isolate the organism by blood and tissue cultures are made. Management is predominantly medical, with adequate duration of appropriate antibiotics.

Spinal tuberculosis accounts for more than 90% of chronic pediatric spinal infections and is caused by *Mycobacterium tuberculosis*. Tubercular infections in children can lead to significant vertebral destruction with the risks of deformity development and progression. Children need periodic follow-up until the completion of their growth. With the availability of antitubercular drugs, the outcomes of tuberculosis of the spine have dramatically improved. Uncomplicated tuberculosis of the spine is a medical disease treated well with antitubercular chemotherapy. Pan-vertebral lesions, the risk or presence of a severe deformity, a severe or progressively worsening neurologic deficit, and lack of improvement or deterioration despite adequate chemotherapy are indications for surgery.

Pearls

- Spinal infection in children is a serious medical condition in which early diagnosis and treatment is critical for a successful outcome.
- In early stages without significant destruction, appropriate antimicrobial chemotherapy is the key to a successful outcome.
- In children with spinal tuberculosis, extensive abscess formation and vertebral destruction is common because of the cartilaginous nature of the vertebral bone. But unless vertebral instability is present, these lesions heal well with chemotherapy, obviating the need for surgery in most situations.
- Children with spine-at-risk radiological signs need spinal stabilization to avoid the development of kyphotic deformity.

Pitfalls

- Atypical clinical presentations, including nonspecific fever, malaise, guarded gait, difficulty in walking, and abdominal pain, are common in pediatric diskitis. A thorough history and clinical examination is essential to diagnose spinal infections.
- Although blood parameters to diagnose infection are nonspecific, MRI is the best modality to help pinpoint the diagnosis.
- Posttubercular kyphotic deformity in children is a dynamic deformity that can worsen or improve with growth. Hence, children need continued follow-up until the completion of their growth.
- Isolating the causative organism is the most important element in achieving a successful outcome in children with pyogenic spondylodiskitis. Hence, blood culture, urine culture, and tissue biopsy should be performed to identify the organism.

References

Five Must-Read References

1. Digby JM, Kersley JB. Pyogenic non-tuberculous spinal infection: an analysis of thirty cases. J Bone Joint Surg Br 1979;61:47–55

2. Fernandez M, Carrol CL, Baker CJ. Discitis and vertebral osteomyelitis in children: an 18-year review. Pediatrics 2000;105:1299–1304

3. Chandrasenan J, Klezl Z, Bommireddy R, Calthorpe D. Spondylodiscitis in children: a retrospective series. J Bone Joint Surg Br 2011;93:1122–1125

4. Sobottke R, Seifert H, Fätkenheuer G, Schmidt M, Gossmann A, Eysel P. Current diagnosis and treatment of spondylodiscitis. Dtsch Arztebl Int 2008;105:181–187

5. Gouliouris T, Aliyu SH, Brown NM Spondylodiscitis: update on diagnosis and management. J Antimicrob Chemother 2010;65(Suppl 3):11–24

6. Hayes AJ, Choksey M, Barnes N, Sparrow OC. Spinal tuberculosis in developed countries: difficulties in diagnosis. J R Coll Surg Edinb 1996;41:192–196

7. Jain AK, Kumar J. Tuberculosis of spine: neurological deficit. Eur Spine J 2013;22(Suppl 4):624–633

8. Rajasekaran S, Prasad Shetty A, Dheenadhayalan J, Shashidhar Reddy J, Naresh-Babu J, Kishen T. Morphological changes during growth in healed childhood spinal tuberculosis: a 15-year prospective study of 61 children treated with ambulatory chemotherapy. J Pediatr Orthop 2006;26:716–724

9. Rajasekaran S. The natural history of post-tubercular kyphosis in children. Radiological signs which predict late increase in deformity. J Bone Joint Surg Br 2001;83:954–962

Infectious Lesions in the Craniovertebral Junction (Suboccipital Region)

Alexander Yu. Mushkin and Alexander V. Gubin

Introduction

The term *suboccipital region* is used to denote the area formed by the occipital condyles, upper cervical vertebrae-C1 and C2, cranio-cervical ligaments, and joints, including the craniovertebral joints (atlanto-occipital joint, median atlantoaxial joint [Cruveilhier's joint], and lateral atlantoaxial joints). Its peculiar anatomy is a unique part of the human skeleton that provides functional support and high mobility of the head, while protecting the elements of the central nervous system and large vascular formations.

Infectious lesions in this region are also unique in their presentation and management. Infection may affect simultaneously the articulations of the occipital bone with the atlas from one or both sides, and the articulations of the atlas with the axis or the bones per se. Destruction of any element of this unified anatomic and functional system has an impact on the entire region and results in atlanto-occipital or atlantoaxial instability and subluxation, including basilar impression. The proximity of the medulla oblongata and cranial parts of the spinal cord determine the risk of neurologic complications that may be life threatening.

Early diagnosis and appropriate treatment are of paramount importance to prevent the development of potential life-threatening complications. As in osteomyelitic lesions of other locations, infection in the suboccipital region may be caused by specific bacterial flora, tuberculosis, or mycotic agents.[1-7] These infections can occur de novo or may be associated with a compromised immune system as well as with the pathology of the oral cavity or from the adjacent ear, nasal, and pharyngeal regions.[5,8,9]

Tuberculosis of the craniovertebral junction (CVJ) has been more commonly reported than other infective organisms.[1-4,6,7,9] Tuberculosis in the suboccipital region is one of the rarest and most severe conditions in bones and joints; it occurs in only 0.3 to 1.0% of patients with tuberculosis spondylitis.[2,10-18] Similar to osseous tuberculous lesions in other parts of the body, suboccipital lesion can be associated with other locations of tuberculosis (commonly from the lungs, gastrointestinal viscera, kidneys, and lymph nodes) with an incidence ranging from 3 to 41%.[16]

Clinical Manifestations and Complications

The specific features and clinical manifestations of craniovertebral (suboccipital) osteomyelitis depend on the anatomic peculiarities of the

Table 12.1 Pathological Syndromes Detected by Infectious Lesions in the Suboccipital Area

Pathological Syndrome	Specific Manifestations
Inflammation due to infection	*Clinical signs*: fever, constitutional symptoms, local neck swelling (anterior and posterior parts), difficulty in breathing, signs of sepsis *Laboratory tests*: elevated CRP, ESR, procalcitonin, and others *Image findings*: bone destruction, abscesses, edema (MRI)
Destruction of stabilising structures of cervical bone	*Clinical signs*: neck motion restriction, stiff neck, head tilt, relief of symptoms by manual or neck brace support of the head *Image findings*: deformities (torticollis), dislocations (subluxation and dislocation) in the Oc-C1-C2 area
Mechanical instability	*Clinical signs*: neck pain, pain in the back of the neck *Image findings*: dislocations in Oc-C1-C2 segments, spinal canal stenosis in the craniovertebral region, axial shift of C2 dens
Neurologic instability	*Clinical signs*: paresis, paralysis, disorder of breathing and swallowing *Image findings*: compression of the lower parts of the medulla oblongata and upper parts of the spinal cord by an abscess, dislocated vertebras or bone fragments; myelopathy (changes in the spinal cord structure)

Abbreviations: CRP, C-reactive protein; ESR, erythrocyte sedimentation rate; Oc, occiput.

affected zone and the etiology of the infection (**Table 12.1**). Upper neck pain and occipital pain, which sometimes can be described as occipital neuralgia, are usually present, and the pain is typically worsened by movements of the head, especially by rotation and bending. In cases of suboccipital tuberculosis, axial neck pain is present in 98%, stiffness of the neck muscles in 82%, and dysphagia due to prevertebral abscesses in 77%.[16] Rarely, submandibular swelling can be evident due to retropharyngeal abscesses. General inflammatory symptoms, such as fever, sepsis, and weakness, are more characteristic of acute nonspecific osteomyelitis, whereas in granulomatous infections the symptoms are malaise, weight loss, and loss of appetite.

Severe neurologic complications, such as complete or incomplete quadriplegia, dyspnea, are rare due to the large reserved space for the spinal cord in the craniocervical spinal canal. These complications can rarely result from large epidural abscesses that compress the spinal cord or the caudal part of the medulla oblongata along with cranio-cervical instability.

The assessment of functional dependence or disability is of importance in deciding the choice of treatment (conservative a or combination of conservative and surgical methods) and in achieving a successful outcome. The grades of disability in suboccipital osteomyelitis are as follows: grade I, moderate cervical pain and complete independence; grade II, limited disability and preserved functional motion and breathing ability; grade III, partial dependence on assistance; grade IV, complete dependence on assistance, with severe myelopathy and breathing difficulties.[4,6,10,15,19]

◾ Imaging Methods

Given the specific anatomy of the suboccipital region, plain films (**Fig. 12.1a,b**), which were generally used in the past, are currently used only for a preliminary analysis of the pathology. The main visualization methods are computed tomography (CT) (**Fig. 12.1c–f**) and magnetic resonance imaging (MRI) (**Fig. 12.1g,h**).

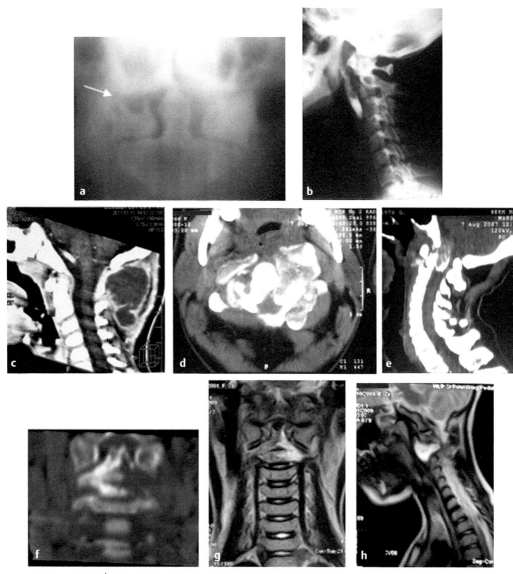

Fig. 12.1 Imaging of suboccipital osteomyelitis in different case scenario. **(a)** Tuberculosis (TB) of the right craniovertebral junction (CVJ) in a 48-year old woman. A radiographic tomogram (coronal section) shows destruction of the upper part of C1 right lateral mass; **(b)** abscess descends to the C3-C4 disk level (contrast introduced after puncturing the lateral neck surface). Nonspecific osteomyelitis of the posterior C1 arch (sagittal computed tomography [CT] scan) in a 6-year old boy: **(c)** an extensive posterior abscess between the occipital bone and the C4 arch. TB of the occiput–C2 in a 58-year-old man: **(d,e)** extensive calcified pre-/retrovertebral and epidural abscesses as observed in the axial **(d)** and sagittal **(e)** CT images. Nonspecific osteomyelitis of the left half of C2 body and dens in a 5-year-old girl: **(f)** bone destruction in the coronal CT is present and **(g,h)** magnetic resonance imaging (MRI) shows prevertebral (retropharyngeal) abscess with a nonhomogeneous content.

Because of the complex osseous anatomy of the craniovertebral junction, CT is ordered with a low threshold in patients with suspected CVJ infection. Multiplane CT reconstructions including three-dimensional (3D) CT are highly informative not only for visualization of the bony structures of the craniovertebral zone, but also for detailing the features of destruction (superficial, focal, or subtotal) and their sequelae, including atlas-occipital or atlantoaxial dislocations. Destruction of the lateral atlas mass has been noted to occur in 48% of suboccipital tuberculosis cases and C1-C2 subluxation in 68%.[16] Asymmetric bone lesions and irregular destruction are typical for osteomyelitis (in contrast with rheumatoid arthritis). The abscesses can be diagnosed on CT based on the widening of the prevertebral (retropharyngeal) tissues and epidural masses.

Magnetic resonance imaging is the method of choice for visualizing soft tissue, the changes in the spinal cord, the structure of the abscesses, and their extension. MRI is highly useful for early diagnosis of inflammatory bone marrow edema and arthritis, but it is less informative for detailed analysis of bone destruction when compared with CT.

Positron emission tomography (PET) CT aids in diagnosis, in particular when the process is of a slow course and with minimal destruction, but it does not help in differentiating between an inflammatory cause and an infectious process.[5]

Magnetic resonance imaging and angio-CT aid in visualizing the vertebral artery and its involvement by abscesses or soft tissue inflammation, which is important in decreasing the risk of damaging the artery during surgery.

Differential Diagnosis

Infectious lesions in the craniovertebral junction need to be differentiated from other destructive processes, in particular from a noninfectious inflammation and tumors in this region.

Noninfectious Inflammation

The craniovertebral region may be affected by rheumatoid arthritis (RA). Clinical features associated with RA are limitation of rotation and torticollis due to pain. Radiological investigation reveals swelling in the region of the joints and hypertrophy of the synovial pannus. If the disease is of long duration, erosion of the joint surfaces and even destruction of bones that form the Cruveilhier's joint may occur (**Fig. 12.2a,b**). In contrast with infectious lesions, soft tissue fluid collections are not characteristic for RA.

Tumors in the Craniovertebral Junction

Infectious spondylitis should first be differentiated from tumors that grow extravertebrally. Their radiographic picture may look similar to that of a paravertebral or epidural abscess. Such changes are frequently noted in chordomas and chondrosarcomas of the clivus and upper cervical vertebrae (**Fig. 12.2c,d**), and more rarely by metastasis of other tumors. Due to a radiological image similarity, suboccipital infections in children should be differentiated from systemic lytic lesions such as histiocytosis (**Fig. 12.2e**).

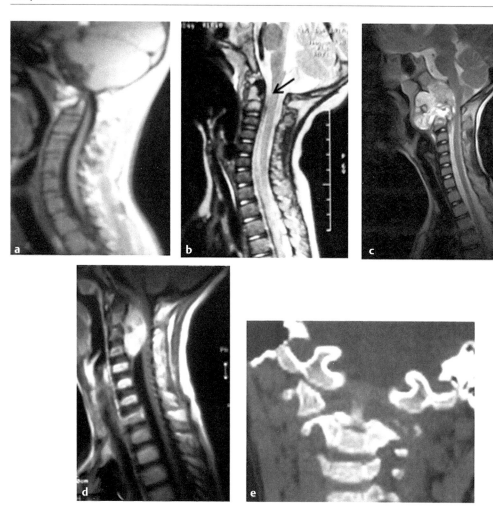

Fig. 12.2 MRI and CT scans of the craniovertebral junction in different destructive processes. Rheumatoid arthritis in a 27-year-old patient under prolonged hormonal therapy: **(a)** C2 dens destruction, swelling of the axial Cruveilhier's joint, and stenosis of the spinal canal in the CVJ; **(b)** hypertrophy of the pannus *(arrow)* in rheumatoid arthritis (RA). Chondrosarcoma of the clivus in a 6-year old girl: **(c)** sagittal MRI showing an extensive heterogenous signal intensity mass involving the clivus, C1 and C2. **(d)** Upper cervical metastasis of a rhabdoid tumor in a 9-year-old boy. **(e)** CT showing destruction of the left lateral C1 mass in a 4-year-old boy with Langerhans cell histiocytosis.

Diagnosis

Etiologic confirmation is mandatory for administration of adequate antibacterial therapy to arrest the infectious process. Puncture/aspiration biopsy of the abscess is done to harvest the material for detection of infection agents. Optimal approaches for the puncture are as follows: transoral approach if the abscess is extended prevertebrally and retropharyngeally; lateral cervical approach if the abscess spreads along the lateral neck surface; the posterior approach in posterior spondylitis if the abscess involves the occipital and suboccipital regions. For the posterior approach, one may need to use CT or the image intensifier to acquire the tissue. In cases where the abscess content is composed of granuloma or necrotic tissues, the biopsy should be performed in an open manner.

Tissue microscopy, culture of the isolated tissue, and modern molecular and genetic methods (polymerase chain reaction, detection of mutated genes that are responsible for bacterial resistance to pharmaceutical drugs) are used to detect infectious agents. Due to the fact that the processes of granulomatosis osteomyelitis of different etiology have similar morphological features, special methods of staining are used for visualization of bacteria and fungi (Ziehl-Neelsen, Grocott, and some others).

Treatment Methods

Management of infectious lesions in the craniovertebral region includes appropriate antibiotic therapy along with management of vertebral lesions.

Antimicrobial therapy is administered taking into consideration the infectious agents and their sensitivity to antibacterial preparations. Antimicrobial therapy should be administered as follows:

- Initially antibiotics are administered intravenously followed by oral antibiotics.
- For a duration not less than 12 months in patients with tuberculosis. The regimens

and the set of antibacterial preparations is based on the World Health Organization guidelines or other established recommendations that take into account the features of sensitivity of the mycobacteria.
- For a duration not less than 6 months in patients with mycosis. The choice of the preparation depends on the type of fungus.

In cases in which the disease process developed on a background of either secondary immunodeficiency (such as human immunodeficiency virus [HIV]) or primary immunodeficiency (PID, e.g., chronic granulomatous disease), antibacterial preparations can be administered throughout life and combined with antiretroviral therapy for HIV or immune replacement medication for PID. Rest and chemotherapy seem to be sufficient for clinical recovery if neurologic and orthopedic complications are absent.[1,3,7,10,20]

Orthotic Application

Orthoses should be used that provide fixation for the upper part of the chest with padded supports for the lower jaw and occipital plate. (four-point cervical collar or Philadelphia-type brace).

Temporary Fixation Devices

In urgent cases or for preparation to surgery, the halo vest can be effective for temporary fixation (**Fig. 12.3**) that provides sufficient stability to the neck.[4]

Surgical Treatment

Table 12.2 lists the indications for surgical treatment of infectious lesions in the craniovertebral junction area.

Currently, surgical treatment is regarded as the method of choice for lesions that are accompanied by marked disability (grades III and IV).[6,10] Removal of abscesses and destructed bone tissue can be performed from the transoral or lateral submandibular approach, and results in a positive effect in the majority of

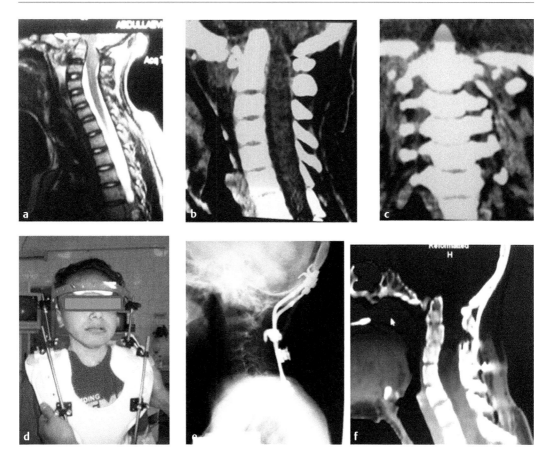

Fig. 12.3 Tuberculosis spondylitis with C1 destruction in an 8-year-old girl with generalized TB and primary immunodeficiency (chronic granulomatous disease). **(a–c)** Total destruction of the C1 lateral masses resulted in C2 dens displacement into the foramen magnum (C2 inclination) and neurologic (motor and breathing) impairment. **(d)** Urgent application of the halo vest with a minimum axial distraction led to a complete relief of neurologic symptoms for several hours. **(e)** Only posterior instrumentation was performed. Although the patient received nonspecific antibacterial and antituberculosis therapy for 8 years, new TB foci developed (lymphatic nodes, soft tissues of the thigh), but there is no recurrence of suboccipital TB, and the patient's neurologic status shows no impairment. She is functionally completely independent. **(f)** CT revealed degeneration of the disks and a partial vertebral block in the zone of fixation by maintenance of C2 dens cranial inclination.

Table 12.2 Indications for Surgical Treatment

Complications	Surgical Intervention
Destruction, abscess	Abscess puncture, debridement
Instability in Oc-C1, C1-C2, Oc-C1-C2; dislocation including C2 dens inclination; deformity	Temporary fixation with halo-cast fixation with posterior instrumentation, occipitospondylodesis (bony)
Spinal cord compression, medulla oblongata compression	Anterior decompression or posterior decompression and stabilization

cases.[8,21] Acute reduction of gross dislocations in this region is not only difficult but also extremely dangerous.[22] To prevent complications associated with the change of the patient's head position during the operation, the intervention may be performed with the halo vest in place for fixation (**Fig. 12.4**), or performed immediately after fixation with posterior instrumentation.[4]

Fixation with posterior instrumentation can be performed as an addition to the removal of pathological tissues or as an independent intervention that provides clinical improvement due to the stability of the craniovertebral junction thus achieved.[4,6,9] Extension of instrumentation is defined by the lesion zone. In an isolated craniovertebral destruction, it may be limited by the zone of the occiput to C2. If the C2 vertebra is involved into the process, the lower fixation level may be extended in the caudal direction (**Fig. 12.5**).

Our own clinical experience of long-term follow-up after the interventions in actively growing children has shown that an excessive extension of instrumentation can result in secondary degenerative changes of the initially unaffected segments in the subaxial spine even if the clinical effects were good (**Fig. 12.3e**).

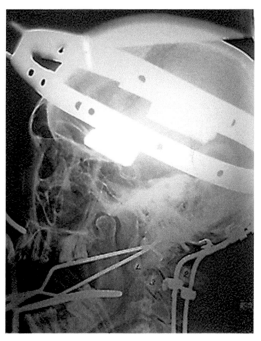

Fig. 12.4 Intraoperative radiograph of a 58-year-old man with suboccipital TB spondylitis (initial patient's findings are shown in **Fig. 12.1d,e**). With the halo cast in place, posterior craniovertebral instrumentation was performed followed by the debridement of the pathological masses via the transoral approach, and anterior spinal cord decompression was performed under the same anesthesia (curettes are positioned in the epidural abscess).

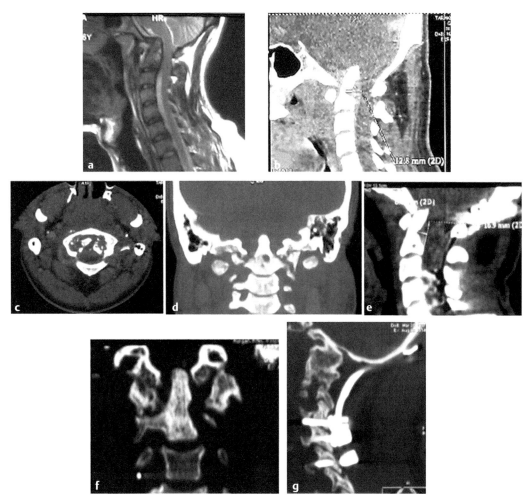

Fig. 12.5 Nonspecific occiput-C1-C2 osteomyelitis in a 52-year-old man. **(a)** Preoperative MRI and **(b–d)** CT scans show destruction of both lateral C1 masses and occipital condyles. The destruction focus is at the C2 dens, with an epidural abscess. Multiple sequestrated bone fragments are seen, and the C2 dens is displaced into the foramen magnum, but spinal cord stenosis is absent. The patient complained of severe pain, forced head position, and fever. There were no neurologic symptoms. Posterior craniovertebral instrumentation (occiput–C5) was performed, which resulted in a significant reduction in **(e)** C2 displacement immediately after the operation and partial bone restoration. **(f,g)** Occiput-C1 ankylosis (fusion) at 1-year follow-up.

Chapter Summary

Osteomyelitis of the craniovertebral junction is a rare life-threatening condition. Due to the unique anatomy of the C0-C1-C2 area, the destructive changes of osteomyelitis frequently result in instability and neurologic symptoms. Severe pain, sharp limitation of neck movements or torticollis along with inflammation, fever, and neck swelling are the characteristic clinical manifestations. Osteomyelitis is often accompanied by swallowing difficulties and sometimes by rapid development of a neurologic deficit. CT and MRI are useful to detect compression of the lower parts of the medulla oblongata and upper spinal cord caused by an abscess and displaced vertebras or bone fragments along with myelopathy. Infectious lesions of the craniovertebral junction should be differentiated from other destructive lesions, such as noninfectious inflammation or neoplasms in this area. Etiologic confirmation is mandatory to administer an adequate antibacterial therapy. Puncture biopsy is commonly used. Optimal approaches for biopsy are the transoral, lateral neck, or posterior approaches. The causative infectious agents are identified by microscopy, culture study, and molecular genetics methods. Once the infection agent is verified and its sensitivity is confirmed, chemotherapy is administered for not less than 6 weeks in nonspecific infections and for not less than for 12 months in tuberculosis. In mycosis, the therapy continues for not less than 6 months. Abscesses and destructed bone tissue are removed from either the transoral or lateral submandibular approach, which is effective in most cases. To prevent complications associated with the change of the head position during the surgery, interventions are performed with the halo cast in place or it may be applied immediately after the posterior instrumentation.

Pearls

- Severe axial neck pain, sharp restriction of neck motion or torticollis along with inflammation, fever, and neck swelling are the characteristic clinical manifestations of CVJ osteomyelitis.
- Etiologic confirmation is mandatory for rational targeted antibacterial therapy. Puncture biopsy is commonly used for acquiring the tissue.
- Transoral, lateral submandibular, and posterior approaches are useful for debridement in CVJ osteomyelitis.
- A halo vest can be used to prevent an abnormal head position after surgery or dangerous head motion during surgery.
- Posterior craniovertebral instrumentation is the best solution for continuous stability in occiput-C1-C2 osteomyelitis.

Pitfalls

- Do not assign antibiotic therapy without bacteriological confirmation of the diagnosis.
- In the presence of craniovertebral instability, do not limit the surgery only to debridement; stable fixation is mandatory.
- Do not cease the course of antibacterial therapy based on clinical symptoms alone in craniovertebral osteomyelitis. Therapy should be for not less than 6 weeks for nonspecific osteomyelitis and for not less than 12 months for tuberculosis caused by drug-sensitive *Mycobacterium* (including a 4-month intensive course) and for not less than 18 months for tuberculosis caused by multidrug-resistant *Mycobacterium* (including a 6-month intensive course).

References

Five Must-Read References

1. Hoshino C, Narita M. Craniovertebral junction tuberculosis: a case report and review of the literature. J Infect Chemother 2010;16:288–291
2. Lavrov VN, Kiselev AM. Treatment policy for craniovertebral spondylitis. Probl Tuberk Bolezn Legk 2007;8:53-61. [in Russian]
3. Mohindra S, Gupta SK, Mohindra S, Gupta R. Unusual presentations of craniovertebral junction tuberculosis: a report of 2 cases and literature review. Surg Neurol 2006;66:94–99, discussion 99
4. Mushkin AIu, Sovetova NA, Alatortsev AV, et al. [Suboccipital tuberculosis: the clinical and radiation and potentialities of current surgical treatment]. [in Russian]. Probl Tuberk Bolezn Legk 2008; 12:40–45
5. Nomura M, Shin M, Ohta M, Nukui Y, Ohkusu K, Saito N. Atypical osteomyelitis of the skull base and craniovertebral junction caused by Actinomyces infection—case report. Neurol Med Chir (Tokyo) 2011;51:64–66
6. Mehrotra A, Das KK, Nair AP, et al. Pediatric craniovertebral junction tuberculosis: management and outcome. Childs Nerv Syst 2013;29:809–814
7. Appaduray SP, Lo P. Nonoperative management of craniovertebral junction and cutaneous tuberculosis. Surg Neurol Int 2015;6:157

8. Ducic Y. Management of osteomyelitis of the anterior skull base and craniovertebral junction. Otolaryngol Head Neck Surg 2003;128):39–42

9. Mushkin AYu, Vishnevsky AA, Burlakov SV. Upper cervical spine tuberculosis spondylitis in patient with HIV infection. [in Russian]. Neurochirurgiya. 2015;2: 68–72

10. Behari S, Nayak SR, Bhargava V, Banerji D, Chhabra DK, Jain VK. Craniocervical tuberculosis: protocol of surgical management. Neurosurgery 2003;52:72–80, discussion 80–81

11. Ibahioin K, Ait Ben Ali A, Choukri M, et al. [Suboccipital tuberculosis: a case report]. Neurochirurgie 2001;47:66–68

12. Grancea V. For X-ray diagnosis of suboc cipital area. Radiol Diagn (Berl) 1960;5:675–687

13. Ousehal A, Gharbi A, Zamiati W, Saidi A, Kadiri R. [Imaging findings in 122 cases of Pott's disease]. Neurochirurgie 2002;48:409–418

14. Pandya SK. Tuberculous atlanto-axial dislocation (with remarks on the mechanism of dislocation). Neurol India 1971;19:116–121

15. Karapurkar AP. Tuberculous atlanto-axial disease including dislocation. NIMHANS J 1988;6(Suppl):89–98

16. Stecken J, Boissonnet H, Manzo L, Pheline C, Dobbelaere P, Yaffi D. [Suboccipital Pott's disease]. Neurochirurgie 1987;33:482–486

17. Krishnan A, Patkar D, Patankar T, et al. Craniovertebral junction tuberculosis: a review of 29 cases. J Comput Assist Tomogr 2001;25:171–176

18. Tuli SM, Rajasekaran S. Tuberculosis of the Skeletal System (Bones, Joints, Spine and Bursal Sheaths), 5th ed. New Delhi: Jaypee Brothers Medical Publishers; 2016:412

19. Lifeso R. Atlanto-axial tuberculosis in adults. J Bone Joint Surg Br 1987;69:183–187

20. Chadha M, Agarwal A, Singh AP. Craniovertebral tuberculosis: a retrospective review of 13 cases managed conservatively. Spine 2007;32:1629–1634

21. Wang LX. Peroral focal debridement for treatment of tuberculosis of the atlas and axis. Chir J Orthop 1981; 1:207–209

22. Fang D, Leong JCY, Fang HSY. Tuberculosis of the upper cervical spine. J Bone Joint Surg Br 1983;65:47–50

13

Minimally Invasive Surgery in Spinal Infections

Moritz Perrech and Roger Hartl

Introduction

Minimally invasive surgery (MIS) of spinal disorders consists of procedures that aim at reducing the extent of the approach to cause less collateral tissue damage, decrease procedure-related morbidity, and achieve more rapid functional recovery without changing the intended surgical goal.[1] In the lumbar spine, these aims can often be achieved by three major surgical techniques: a unilateral MIS approach for "over the top" contralateral decompression; minimizing instability using undercutting of spinal anatomy, rather than open surgery, and resection of stabilizing structures; and indirect decompression by implantation of interbody cages. Although the first two techniques are also suitable for the minimally invasive treatment of spinal infections, the third technique is rarely applicable.

Eradication of the underlying infection, restoration of spinal integrity, recovery from neurologic deficits, and pain therapy are the main principles of surgical treatment of spinal infections.[2,3] The goals of surgical treatment are removal of the septic focus, acquisition of a specimen for microbiological workup, decompression of neuronal structures, and stabilization as well as restoration of the affected spinal segments[4] (**Table 13.1**).

In selected cases, MIS techniques can be used to achieve the surgical goals for the treatment of spinal infections. This is of the highest importance, as patients with spinal infections often suffer from a broad range of medical disorders. In recent years, several studies have been published on MIS strategies for the treatment of spinal infections. Among these strategies are tubular or extreme lateral approaches to the spine, and endoscopic and transpedicular techniques. Additionally, there is increasing

Table 13.1 Indications for Surgery in Spinal Infections

Pyogenous vertebral osteomyelitis
Progressive neurologic deficit
Progressive deformity
Spinal instability
Therapy-refractory pain
Additional intraspinal abscess (see below)
Failed conservative treatment
Recurrent bloodstream infection
Unclear etiology of the process
Granulomatous vertebral osteomyelitis (e.g., tuberculosis)
Neurologic deficit
Spinal cord compression (> 50%)
Long segment disease (> 4 vertebrae)
Kyphosis > 60 degrees
Large abscess (paraspinal or epidural)
Severe pain
Spinal epidural abscess
Neurologic deficit
Severe clinical signs of infection

interest in percutaneous navigation-guided techniques for the safe and less invasive instrumentation of the affected spinal segments.

Overview of Different Minimally Invasive Techniques

In general, the goals of minimally invasive techniques are a decrease in morbidity and a faster functional recovery by reducing collateral tissue damage through less extensive approaches and by using preformed anatomic corridors.[1] In accordance with AO Spine principles, the goals of minimally invasive treatment of spinal infections are (1) stabilization of pathological instability, (2) restoration of spinal balance, (3) preservation of neurologic function, and (4) administration of appropriate chemotherapy.[5] Based on these principles, there is a multitude of MIS techniques for the treatment of spinal infections using anterior, posterior, and endoscopic approaches (**Table 13.2**). The choice

Table 13.2 Overview of Minimally Invasive Techniques Used in the Treatment of Spinal Infections

Anterior/lateral approaches
ALIF
XLIF
MIS DLIF
Posterior approaches
MIS TLIF
Transpedicular curettage
Endoscopic approaches
Endoscopic diskectomy (PED)
Endoscopic abscess drainage
Thoracoscopy (VATS)
Screw insertion techniques
Intraoperative navigation
Robot-assisted screw placement

Abbreviations: ALIF, anterior lumbar interbody fusion; DLIF, direct lateral interbody fusion; MIS, minimally invasive surgery; PED, percutaneous endoscopic debridement; TLIF, transforaminal lumbar interbody fusion; VATS, video-assisted thoracoscopic surgery; XLIF, extreme lateral interbody fusion.

of the approach should be tailored to the site, the morphology, and the extent and etiology of the pathology. For example, cervical infections are often primarily managed through an anterior approach, endoscopy is widely used for thoracic lesions. In contrast, lumbar infections are often treated posteriorly. More severe infections may require combined approaches or even a 360-degree fusion.

Anterior/Lateral Techniques

Anterior approaches to the spine provide direct access to the most common sites of infection—the vertebral body and the intervertebral disk. Additionally, in cases of a secondary severe deformity, anterior approaches are often required to restore spinal balance and integrity. However, anterior approaches are associated with a significant procedure-related morbidity, particularly in the thoracic and lumbar spine. Therefore, MIS techniques use less extensive approaches (minimally invasive anterior lumbar interbody fusion [ALIF]) or alternative routes to access the anterior column of the spine, such as extreme lateral interbody fusion (XLIF) and direct lateral interbody fusion (DLIF). The literature on the effectiveness of these approaches for the treatment of spinal infections is scarce. However, recently MIS lateral accesses to the anterior vertebral column have gained an increasing interest for the treatment of lumbar degenerative pathologies. Consequently, similar approaches have now been applied for the surgical treatment of spinal infections. In their case series, Lee at al[6] retrospectively analyzed the morbidity and clinical outcomes of patients with infectious spondylitis treated with minimal-access lateral approaches compared with traditional anterior approaches. The authors reported a high fusion rate of 97% for both groups and a lower complication rate for the minimal-access group. In 2015, Blizzard et al[7] and Patel at al[8] published the results of their case series, in which they used an extreme lateral approach for the treatment of spondylodiskitis (specifically XLIF).[7,8] Based on their experiences, they concluded that XLIF may be a

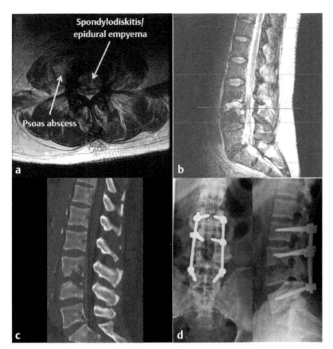

Fig. 13.1 Illustrative case 1: a 69-year-old patient presents with severe lower back pain and acute weakness in both legs. **(a,b)** Preoperative magnetic resonance imaging (MRI) shows spondylodiskitis in L3-L4 with epidural empyema and right-sided psoas abscess. **(c)** Computed tomography (CT) shows partial destruction of adjacent vertebral bodies. **(d)** First, open posterior fixation was performed from L2 to L5.

safe and effective technique for the treatment of spondylitis. However, it has to be noted that the studies published to date are limited because of small numbers of patients and the lack of information about complications. Nevertheless, these are promising results for the use of MIS techniques in the treatment of spondylitis. The techniques offer sufficiently wide access to the anterior spine while sparing the posterior elements, in particular the erector spinae muscles. This helps reduce the tissue trauma, decrease the blood loss and reduce the operative time, which may be particularly beneficial in a population often presenting in poor medical condition.

In line with the current literature, we recommend adding posterior fixation after lateral or anterior approaches to the spine in patients with spondylitis, as this facilitates early mobilization of patients. The addition of a lateral plate to avoid a posterior fixation may not offer sufficient mechanical support to enable mobilization. Intraoperatively, care should be taken not to violate the end plates to limit cage subsidence. The lateral MIS approach to the spine may also be used to remove adjacent psoas abscesses (**Figs. 13.1** and **13.2**).

Posterior Techniques

Posterior approaches to the spine are commonly used for a multitude of indications. Therefore, many spine surgeons feel comfortable with these approaches when treating spinal infections. Among others, posterior techniques used for the treatment of spinal infections consist of posterior or posterolateral interbody fusion, simple decompressions with or without additional instrumentation, transforaminal interbody fusion (TLIF), and transpedicular curettage. All of these techniques and variations can be used as minimally invasive techniques.

Simple decompressions can be performed with minimally invasive techniques similar to previously published techniques for microdiskectomy or spinal decompression through a tubular retractor. In our experience, minimally invasive decompression is a valuable treatment option, particularly in spinal epidural abscesses, where the removal of intraspinal empyema can be performed even in multilevel pathologies. To date, there are no larger studies that provide evidence that this technique is effective in the treatment of spinal infections. However, a few case series have been published

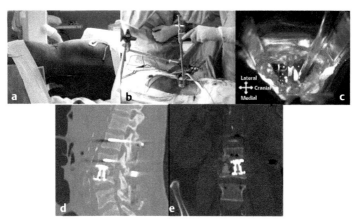

Fig. 13.2 Illustrative case 1, continued. Intra- and postoperative images. **(a)** The patient was placed in the lateral position. **(b)** With intraoperative monitoring a transmuscular approach was performed. **(c)** En route, the psoas abscess was removed from the left side along the retroperitoneal route. After wide removal of lytic bone tissue, an expandable cage was implanted. Postoperative CT scan shows a good cage position and improved lumbar lordosis. **(d,e)** The implanted cage is supported by the intact part of the L3 end plate and the intact L4 end plate.

that show successful treatment of spinal epidural abscess through a minimally invasive tubular approach.[9] The question of whether minimally invasive decompression alone is sufficient for the treatment of spondylitis remains unanswered. Although some authors recommend using additional posterior instrumentation, others refrain from that in fear of an increased re-infection rate due to superinfection of implanted instrumentation material. In case of spondylitis, we usually recommend adding posterior instrumentation because, in our experience, the re-infection rates are low and the additional instrumentation facilitates the early mobilization of patients.

Another minimally invasive technique that is commonly applied in the treatment of lumbar degenerative disorders is TLIF. This technique was first reported by Foley et al[10] in 2003. Similar techniques have also been applied for the treatment of spinal infections. In their cases series, Shiban et al[11] describe the successful treatment of patients with lumbar spondylodiskitis using a TLIF approach and a TLIF cage for anterior fusion. Whether a titanium or polyetheretherketone (PEEK) cage is used does not seem to influence the outcomes in terms of the re-infection and fusion rates.[12]

In cases of spondylodiskitis without bony destruction, we usually perform an MIS that is similar to TLIF. The same operative goals can be achieved by posterior lumbar interbody fusion (PLIF), which can also be performed in a minimally invasive technique. The more medial approach of a PLIF may facilitate decompression of neuronal structures and a more rigid fixation, as the ipsilateral facet joint is not removed completely. However, in our experience, this approach is often more invasive than the TLIF approach and is associated with a higher risk of accidental durotomy, which can lead to an intradural spreading of infection.

Other less invasive posterior techniques for the treatment of spinal infections have been published. Most of these techniques are applied percutaneously and use a transpedicular approach. In 2014, Lee et al[13] published their results of a retrospective analysis of percutaneous transpedicular curettage and drainage compared with a combined anterior and posterior approach in patients with spondylodiskitis. In their approach, after the placement of pedicle screws in adjacent healthy segments, pedicle holes were drilled in the infected segment. Through this route, the infected space was then rinsed with saline. A drain was left in place for the postoperative period until the amount of drainage was low enough for removal. The authors reported that patients treated with this technique were able to be mobilized earlier than patients who were treated via a combined anterior and posterior approach. However, the intraoperative blood loss was more extensive in the study group, and antibiotics had to be administered for a longer period of time.

The same transpedicular approach has been used by other authors to access the infected disk space for microbiological sampling, removal of infected material, and additional fusion with bone graft.[14] These transpedicular techniques are of limited usefulness in treating cases of more extensive bony destruction or cases of compression of neuronal structures where a more invasive approach may be warranted.

Most spine surgeons refrain from using percutaneous cement augmentation techniques in spinal infections. Even in cases of a de novo spinal deformity due to infectious destruction of bone or intervertebral disk material, vertebroplasty and kyphoplasty of affected segments cannot be recommended. However, augmentation of screws in healthy adjacent segments may be helpful in creating a stable construct, particularly in patients with severe osteoporosis.

Endoscopic Techniques

Endoscopic techniques have been used for the treatment of degenerative disorders of the spine since the 1980s. Subsequently, the indications for these techniques have evolved in many fields of spinal surgery, and endoscopy has also been implemented in the treatment of spinal infections.

Among other techniques, percutaneous endoscopic diskectomy and drainage (PEDD) has been reported as a minimally invasive technique for the treatment of spinal infections. In this technique, the infected disk is accessed with an endoscope percutaneously through a posterolateral approach under fluoroscopic guidance. Tissue sampling and diskectomy are then performed endoscopically followed by irrigation and placement of a drain that is connected to a pump and left in place until the drainage resolves. This technique seems to be particularly effective in tissue sampling, when compared with computed tomography (CT)-guided biopsy, and in the treatment of uncomplicated spondylodiskitis that is limited to the disk space. However, it may be of limited use in more extensive lesions. Another drawback of this technique is the continuous drainage that has to be maintained in the postoperative period, as this may limit the patient's mobilization to a certain degree.[15] Several modifications of this technique have been published such as percutaneous endoscopic debridement with dilute betadine solution irrigation (PEDI), but the same limitations apply as for PEDD.[16]

In more extensive infectious lesions, anterior endoscopic approaches may be indicated. Particularly for the thoracic spine, endoscopic techniques (thoracoscopy) can help reducing the invasiveness of the approach. To date, thoracoscopic approaches have mainly been used for the treatment of tubercular spondylitis. However, there are also a few case reports about its use in the treatment of pyogenous spondylitis. In their case presentation, Détillon et al[17] describe the successful treatment of a bone-destructing infectious lesion of T10-T11 using video-assisted thoracoscopic surgery (VATS). The potential advantages of VATS are a reduction in intraoperative blood loss, earlier mobilization, and shorter postoperative hospital stay when compared with open approaches. However, the technique has limitations in patients who cannot tolerate one-sided ventilation or in cases of severe pleural adhesions.

In cases of a psoas abscess secondary to spondylodiskitis that is refractory to antibiotic treatment, an invasive treatment of the psoas abscess itself may be required. For this indication, endoscopic retroperitoneal approaches (retroperitoneoscopic) have been applied. To render this approach as targeted as possible, laparoscopic ultrasound has been added to precisely detect the site of intramuscular abscess intraoperatively. In comparison to percutaneous

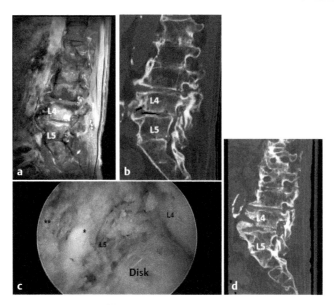

Fig. 13.3 Illustrative case 2: an 86-year-old patient presents with severe lower back pain and bilateral pain in the lower extremities (visual analogue scale [VAS] of leg pain: 6–9/10). Preoperative MRI and CT imaging shows spondylodiskitis in L4-L5 6 months after laminectomies from L2 to S1. **(a,b)** Due to the loss of intervertebral disk height, foraminal stenosis led to bilateral L4 nerve root compression. **(c)** Endo-scopic transforaminal decompression of the L4 nerve root was performed bilaterally. *, yellow ligament of the lateral recess, **, superior articular process. **(d)** Postoperative CT imaging showed decompression of the L4 neuroforamen. The pain level improved significantly (postoperative VAS of leg pain: 2/10).

CT-guided drainage of psoas abscesses, endo-scopic approaches may be particularly valuable in multiloculated abscesses or thick, highly viscous pus.[18]

In cases of loss of disk height due to spondylodiskitis, endoscopic techniques can also be used for the transforaminal decompression of affected nerve roots (**Fig. 13.3**).

Screw Insertion Techniques

Conflicting evidence exists regarding the question of whether instrumentation should be added in infectious spondylitis cases. Although some authors strongly recommend an additional posterior instrumentation as an adjunct to anterior decompression in spinal infections to achieve a higher fusion rate, others refrain from implantation of foreign material due to a potentially increased risk of persistent infection. Moreover, adding instrumentation may prolong the operative time, the intraoperative blood loss, and the procedure-related morbidity. Therefore, as patients with spondylitis often suffer from severe comorbidities, it is of great importance to reduce the invasiveness of the operative treatment. Deininger et al[19] published a case series of 12 patients with spondylodiskitis who were treated by percutaneous posterior instrumentation and a course of antibiotic treatment. After the operation, patients were mobilized on the first postoperative day. No complications occurred, and the patients showed good clinical outcomes in terms of resolution of infection and fusion rates. Nasto et al[20] compared the clinical outcomes of patients with spondylitis who were treated with percutaneous instrumentation with the outcomes of patients who were treated by thoracolumbosacral orthosis (TLSO) as an adjunct to antibiotic treatment. The authors found that the patients treated with percutaneous instrumentation had a faster recovery, lower pain scores, and an improved quality of life.

In the treatment of degenerative spinal diseases, the use of novel technologies, such as navigation, has led to an increased use of percutaneous instrumentation techniques. Navigation techniques have evolved from fluoroscopy to intraoperative imaging and robot-assisted screw placement. These techniques have been shown to increase the accuracy of percutaneous pedicle screw placement. Additionally, in a setting of a well-established spinal navigation, navigation may even help reduce operative times, which is particularly important in patients with multiple comorbidities. Moreover, image guidance for pedicle screw placement may be helpful in an altered anatomy such as in secondary deformities caused by infections.

Tuberculosis

In cases of a spinal manifestation of tuberculosis, usually a primary course of chemotherapeutic treatment is advised. However, there are some indications for surgical treatment (**Table 13.1**).[2,21] Many minimally invasive techniques established for the treatment of spinal degenerative disorders have also been used for the treatment of spinal tuberculosis.

Particularly, VATS has been successfully used for the decompression of the spinal canal and reconstruction of the anterior spinal column in spinal tuberculosis.[22] Moreover, percutaneous pedicle screw instrumentation has been used in combination with transforaminal or lateral approaches to decompress the spinal cord and stabilize the spine.[23] In their study, Garg and

Vohra[24] considered the combination of lateral approaches and percutaneous screw insertion to be a hybrid MIS technique. They found their technique to be as effective in kyphosis correction and preventing secondary spinal deformity as conventional open techniques. Additionally, the complication rate of 9% compared favorably with the complication rates of conventional open approaches (24 to 31%).

There are several limitations to all the studies that analyzed MIS techniques for the treatment of spinal tuberculosis. In particular, the studies are mainly case series that reported outcomes at single centers. However, in selected cases, MIS techniques may be helpful in reducing the approach-related morbidity in patients with spinal tuberculosis.

Chapter Summary

In recent years, MIS techniques have been used increasingly for the treatment of spinal degenerative disorders. Some of these techniques have been used for the treatment of spinal infections as well. These techniques help reduce the approach-related morbidity in a population that often suffers from multiple medical disorders. A broad variety of MIS techniques have been reported for the treatment of spinal infections, some based on endoscopic approaches, and others on transforaminal or lateral approaches. These techniques have been shown to be effective in selected cases; however, most of these studies were case series with low numbers of patients. In our experience, MIS can be a viable option in limited spinal infections with a low degree of end-plate destruction. In addition, percutaneous screw insertion techniques can be safely applied in patients with more severe bone destruction, particularly, with navigated techniques. Due to the lack of evidence, decision making for the use of MIS techniques should be based on a thorough risk-benefit analysis for the individual patient.

- The current limitations of MIS reconstruction have to be clearly understood as they impact the goals of the surgery, namely adequate decompression, stabilization, and restoration of alignment. Thus, it is important to understand that MIS surgery relies largely on indirect decompression of pathology via cages, which in turn requires adequate bone strength and intact end plates. But this requirement is frequently not met in cases of infection. The other principles of MIS surgery are a unilateral approach for bilateral decompression and the minimization of iatrogenic instability by undercutting instead of removing stabilizing structures; these two principles also apply in infection cases.
- If the end plates are affected and destroyed, a pure MIS approach for reconstruction is less likely to be successful.

- Lateral approaches can be effective not only for the treatment of the anterior column of the spine in spinal infections but also to remove intramuscular abscesses of the psoas muscle. However, a posterior percutaneous instrumentation should be added.

- In cases of severe bony destruction with loss of end-plate integrity or in cases of severe compression of the spinal cord, minimally invasive techniques may not be advisable.
- Because MIS techniques involve a steep learning curve, the surgeon must have adequate experience using MIS techniques in degenerative conditions before applying these techniques in patients with infective spondylitis.

References
Five Must-Read References

1. McAfee PC, Phillips FM, Andersson G, et al. Minimally invasive spine surgery. Spine 2010;35(26, Suppl):S271–S273
2. Boody BS, Jenkins TJ, Maslak J, Hsu WK, Patel AA. Vertebral osteomyelitis and spinal epidural abscess: an evidence-based review. J Spinal Disord Tech 2015;28:E316–E327
3. Zarghooni K, Röllinghoff M, Sobottke R, Eysel P. Treatment of spondylodiscitis. Int Orthop 2012;36:405–411
4. Okada Y, Miyamoto H, Uno K, Sumi M. Clinical and radiological outcome of surgery for pyogenic and tuberculous spondylitis: comparisons of surgical techniques and disease types. J Neurosurg Spine 2009;11:620–627
5. Härtl R, Korge A; AOSpine International. Minimally Invasive Spine Surgery: Techniques, Evidence, and Controversies. Davos-Platz, Switzerland: AOSpine; 2012
6. Lee CY, Huang TJ, Li YY, Cheng CC, Wu MH. Comparison of minimal access and traditional anterior spinal surgery in managing infectious spondylitis: a minimum 2-year follow-up. Spine J 2014;14:1099–1105
7. Blizzard DJ, Hills CP, Isaacs RE, Brown CR. Extreme lateral interbody fusion with posterior instrumentation for spondylodiscitis. J Clin Neurosci 2015;22:1758–1761
8. Patel NB, Dodd ZH, Voorhies J, Horn EM. Minimally invasive lateral transpsoas approach for spinal discitis and osteomyelitis. J Clin Neurosci 2015;22:1753–1757
9. Safavi-Abbasi S, Maurer AJ, Rabb CH. Minimally invasive treatment of multilevel spinal epidural abscess. J Neurosurg Spine 2013;18:32–35
10. Foley KT, Holly LT, Schwender JD. Minimally invasive lumbar fusion. Spine 2003; 28(15, Suppl):S26–S35
11. Shiban E, Janssen I, da Cunha PR, et al. Safety and efficacy of polyetheretherketone (PEEK) cages in combination with posterior pedicel screw fixation in pyogenic spinal infection. Acta Neurochir (Wien) 2016;158:1851–1857
12. Schomacher M, Finger T, Koeppen D, et al. Application of titanium and polyetheretherketone cages in the treatment of pyogenic spondylodiscitis. Clin Neurol Neurosurg 2014;127:65–70
13. Lee BH, Park JO, Kim HS, Lee HM, Cho BW, Moon SH. Transpedicular curettage and drainage versus combined anterior and posterior surgery in infectious spondylodiscitis. Indian J Orthop 2014;48:74–80
14. Ikuta K, Masuda K, Yonekura Y, Kitamura T, Senba H, Shidahara S. Percutaneous transpedicular interbody fusion technique in percutaneous pedicle screw stabilization for pseudoarthrosis following pyogenic spondylitis. Asian Spine J 2016;10:343–348
15. Fu TS, Chen LH, Chen WJ. Minimally invasive percutaneous endoscopic discectomy and drainage for infectious spondylodiscitis. Biomed J 2013;36:168–174
16. Yang SC, Fu TS, Chen HS, Kao YH, Yu SW, Tu YK. Minimally invasive endoscopic treatment for lumbar infectious spondylitis: a retrospective study in a tertiary referral center. BMC Musculoskelet Disord 2014;15:105

17. Détillon D, de Groot H, Hoebink E, Versteylen R, Veen E. Video-assisted thoracoscopic surgery as a diagnostic and therapeutic instrument in non-tubercular spondylodiscitis. Int J Spine Surg 2015; 9:55

18. Kodama K, Takase Y, Motoi I, Mizuno H, Goshima K, Sawaguchi T. Retroperitoneoscopic drainage of bilateral psoas abscesses under intraoperative laparoscopic ultrasound guidance. Asian J Endosc Surg 2014;7:179–181

19. Deininger MH, Unfried MI, Vougioukas VI, Hubbe U. Minimally invasive dorsal percutaneous spondylodesis for the treatment of adult pyogenic spondylodiscitis. Acta Neurochir (Wien) 2009;151:1451–1457

20. Nasto LA, Colangelo D, Mazzotta V, et al. Is posterior percutaneous screw-rod instrumentation a safe and effective alternative approach to TLSO rigid bracing for single-level pyogenic spondylodiscitis? Results of a retrospective cohort analysis. Spine J 2014;14: 1139–1146

21. Chandra SP, Singh A, Goyal N, et al. Analysis of changing paradigms of management in 179 patients with spinal tuberculosis over a 12-year period and proposal of a new management algorithm. World Neurosurg 2013;80:190–203

22. Lü G, Wang B, Li J, Liu W, Cheng I. Anterior debridement and reconstruction via thoracoscopy-assisted mini-open approach for the treatment of thoracic spinal tuberculosis: minimum 5-year follow-up. Eur Spine J 2012;21:463–469

23. Kandwal P, Garg B, Upendra B, Chowdhury B, Jayaswal A. Outcome of minimally invasive surgery in the management of tuberculous spondylitis. Indian J Orthop 2012;46:159–164

24. Garg N, Vohra R. Minimally invasive surgical approaches in the management of tuberculosis of the thoracic and lumbar spine. Clin Orthop Relat Res 2014;472:1855–1867

14

Human Immunodeficiency Virus and Spinal Infections

Robert Dunn

Introduction

The human immunodeficiency virus (HIV) has had a dramatic effect on the incidence and effect of spondylodiskitis. By the end of 2015, 36.7 million people globally were living with HIV. During 2015, 2.1 million people had contracted the virus, with 1.1 million dying from it. This disease burden is concentrated in sub-Saharan Africa, which accounts for 25.6 million (70%) of the worldwide HIV-positive population.[1] In this region of the world, a syndemic of HIV and tuberculosis (TB) exists, in which these two diseases converge synergistically to magnify the burden of disease.[2] According to World Health Organization (WHO) data, there were 10.4 million new cases of TB in 2015, of which 1.2 million (11%) were HIV positive. Six countries—India, Indonesia, China, Nigeria, Pakistan, and South Africa—account for 60% of the TB cases. The highest TB/HIV co-infection was in southern Africa. In 2015, there were 1.4 million TB-related deaths, 0.4 million (29%) being HIV positive. The HIV incidence may well be underreported, as only 55% of TB patients worldwide had a documented HIV result, although the numbers are higher in southern Africa, where 81% of TB cases had a recorded HIV status.[3]

The Cellular Impact of HIV and TB

Sexual contact among heterosexuals is the dominant mode of HIV transmission, although outside Africa, a third of cases are due to intravenous drug use. *Mycobacterium tuberculosis* is generally acquired via inhalation. The alveolar macrophages phagocytose the bacilli and process them in transit to the regional lymph node to initiate an adaptive immune response. The bacilli avoid fusion with lysosomes and continue to replicate. An exuberant accumulation of inflammatory cells form a multinucleated giant-cell–rich granuloma within which the bacilli persist.[4] Cell-mediated immunity is essential for control of *M. tuberculosis* infection. Activation of both CD4+ and CD8+ T cells are seen, and CD4+ T lymphocytes of T helper cell type 1(Th1) are thought to be most critical.[5]

Human immunodeficiency virus gains access to cells without immediate lethal damage. It first binds to the CD4 receptor, triggering conformational changes that release the viral core into the cell cytoplasm. The viral genome is reverse transcribed into DNA by the virus's own reverse transcriptase enzyme. This process is error prone, but distinct viral variants may be created. The viral genome is then inserted into gene-rich, transcriptionally active domains of the host's chromosomal DNA, transforming the cell into a potential virus producer. The hallmark of HIV infection is the depletion of CD4+ T cells.[6] This leads to increased TB reactivation. One third of the world's population is thought to be latently infected with *M. tuberculosis,* although the data supporting this notion may be questioned. Approximately 10% of *M. tuberculosis*–infected individuals are thought to develop overt clinical disease, and about half of them develop the disease longer than 2 years after infection. These cases are commonly termed reactivation or postprimary TB. The lifetime risk of developing active TB in immunocompetent adults is estimated to be 5 to 10%, but in HIV-positive individuals this risk is increased to 5 to 15% annually.[5]

Not only does HIV increase the likelihood of TB reactivation, but also TB drives HIV replication by increased HIV-infected CD4+ cell reproduction. Phagocytosis of TB induces macrophage activation and proinflammatory cytokines [tumor necrosis factor-a (TNF-a), interleukin-1β (IL-1β), IL-6], which enhance HIV replication, driving the cycle further.[4]

Clinical Presentation

The commonest general opportunistic infections in HIV+ patients reported from Uganda were candidiasis, diarrhea, geohelminths, TB, malaria, and pneumonia. The candidiasis was confirmed as commonest in an Indian study.[7,8]

In the spine, *M. tuberculosis* remains the overwhelming co-infection. According to unpublished data I have gathered, 69 cases of spondylodiskitis were managed in the 2-year period of 2014–2015 at a single tertiary center base in Cape Town, South Africa; 31 of these cases were confirmed to be HIV positive, of which 26 were due to TB, four to pyogenic bacteria, and one to cryptococcal infection.

Not only does HIV increase the risk of contracting TB, but more importantly there is a 10% annual risk of reactivation as the contained *M. tuberculosis* bacillus is released. This is 12 to 20 times higher than in the immunocompetent individual. HIV also increases the incidence of extrapulmonary TB (EPTB), typically cited in immunocompetent patients as occurring in 10% of cases, half of which are musculoskeletal, the commonest being spinal TB at around 2% of total TB cases.

The clinical presentation is similar to the general presentation of spinal TB in the immunocompetent patient, with delayed presentation due to the insidious nature of the disease, the vague symptoms of pain and weight loss, and the lack of access to health care in the regions of the world where the HIV/TB syndemic exists.

Human immunodeficiency virus is reported as more common in men than in women, with a 2:1 ratio in the age range of 33 to 45 years.[9] This is reversed in southern Africa, where females predominate. This may well be due to woman having a higher risk of contracting HIV when exposed. TB may occur earlier in the HIV course than other opportunistic infections, due to the susceptibility of the *M. tuberculosis*–specific CD4+ cells to HIV and selective TB protective CD4-cell depletion.

Spinal TB may occur in the absence of pulmonary TB. By the time the patients present, there may be clinical kyphotic deformity (gibbus) or even a neurologic deficit. The erythrocyte sedimentation rate (ESR) and C-reactive protein (CRP) are usually raised, with the white cell count being normal.

A study conducted in a first-world hospital with 7,338 HIV-positive admissions in a 6-year period found that the incidence of spinal infection among admitted patients was calculated as 23.2 of 100,000 in the HIV-positive population compared with 7.1 of 100,000 in the HIV-negative population. The authors also found that of the 17 HIV-positive spine infections, eight were pyogenic with a CD4 count average of 339, six had TB with a CD4 count average of 75, and three had epidural abscesses with a CD4 count average of 21.[10]

Diagnosis

Although imaging may be the same as in immunocompetent patients, that is, typically paradiskal kyphotic collapse with preservation of the disk space until later in the infection course, there may be less destruction seen on magnetic resonance imaging (MRI). With moderation of the cell-mediated type 4 hypersensitivity response, there may be less bony destruction and more pus collection.[11] Early disk space height loss with intact bodies suggests pyogenic infection as opposed to the typical paradiskal erosions and kyphosis of *M. tuberculosis* spondylodiskitis.

Magnetic resonance imaging is useful to identify the pathology, determine the abscess size and location, confirm noncontiguous lesions, and assess the spinal cord. Up to 16% of TB spine patients may have noncontiguous vertebral lesions.[12] MRI may confirm an HIV myelitis as a cause of neurologic deterioration rather than any spine infection (**Fig. 14.1**).

Although TB remains by far the commonest infection in the HIV-positive cohort, other infectious or noninfectious causes must be considered, making spinal biopsy mandatory. A positive TB culture is the reference standard for identification of acid-fast bacilli. Microscopy may be negative due to the paucibacillary nature of the infection.

Increasingly, polymerase chain reaction (PCR) technology is utilized, which significantly reduces the 3- to 4-week period required to obtain a culture result. Xpert is a cartridge-based technology used at endemic sites for this very purpose and provides the result immediately. It amplifies a 81 base pair region of *M. tuberculosis* RNA polymerase ß-subunit (rpoß) gene. This is also the site of rifampin resistance, enabling confirmation of this drug's usefulness. In spinal samples, Xpert has a sensitivity and specificity in the 95% range, although some cite it as being 10% lower in HIV-associated disease.

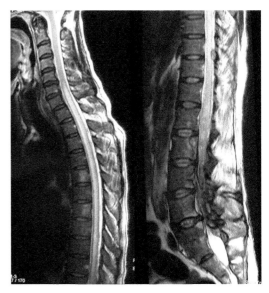

Fig. 14.1 Magnetic resonance imaging (MRI) confirms minimal vertebral involvement with severe cord changes and ascending myelitis, resulting in rapid quadriplegia and subsequent death.

This has not been our experience. As this is genetic material detection, it will be positive even after clinical cure, as it cannot distinguish between live and dead bacillus.[13]

Treatment

Treatment of TB remains the same, irrespective of the HIV status. Due to the socioeconomic factors that make these patients vulnerable to HIV/TB, they are often malnourished and in poor general health. Thus, specific TB and HIV treatment needs to be supported with adequate nutrition and social and educational support.

With regard to TB treatment, first-line management involves combination treatment with rifampin (RIF), isoniazid (isonicotinic acid hydrazide, INH), ethambutol (ETB), and pyrazinamide (PZA). These medications are available in a single preparation to improve compliance. There are a variety of recommendations, with many authors basing their strategy on the pulmonary tuberculosis (PTB) protocol consisting of 2 months of intensive four-drug treatment followed by a continuation phase of RIF/INH for an additional 4 months. In high-burden areas, four-drug treatment is continued for a minimum of 9 months. Although some practitioners may regard this as excessive, there is poor penetration of the drug into large abscesses and bony/diskal debris, which intuitively requires longer courses to avoid recurrence. There is little evidence to support the duration of treatment or the number of drugs, but this is the routine practiced in high-volume centers. The antibiotics are administered using the directly observed treatment, short course (DOTS) protocol, which in South Africa is further incentivized with a financial stipend while on the medical treatment program. Due to the potential peripheral neuropathy from the INH, pyridoxine (vitamin B_6) is added.

Because of the HIV co-infection, cotrimoxazole should be added as prophylaxis against other opportunistic infections such as *Pneumocystis,* isosporiasis, and invasive *Salmonella*; it reduces mortality by up to 46%. It can be discontinued if the CD4 count exceeds 200.[14]

Highly active antiretroviral therapy (HAART) has had great impact on both HIV patients but more specifically on patients with HIV/TB co-infection, with a reduced mortality of 64 to 95%. All co-infected patients should be initiated on HAART. However, the risks of immune reconstitution inflammatory syndrome (IRIS) need to be considered. HIV-infected patients with low CD4+ T-cell counts immunologically tolerate *M. tuberculosis*.[4] As HAART controls the effects of HIV, there is a 10 to 43% incidence of IRIS, where the bolstered immune system is increasingly activated by the *M. tuberculosis*. WHO and South African health authorities recommend a period of anti-TB treatment before initiation of HAART to avoid IRIS. If the CD4 count is less than 50, HAART should be commenced within 2 weeks after TB medication. Where the CD4 count is > 50, the initiation of HAART should be deferred for 8 weeks after initiating anti-TB care.[4,14]

Pre-HAART elevated TNF, high inflammation biomarkers, lower antibodies to phenolic glycolipid (PGL-TB$_1$) antigen, and natural killer cell degranulation levels may predict IRIS. These tests, however, are not readily available where the clinical situation occurs and are expensive.[4]

Should IRIS occur, nonsteroidal anti-inflammatory drugs (NSAIDs) and steroids are the mainstay, and HAART cessation is seldom warranted.[14]

The WHO-recommended HAART in the co-infected patient consists of tenofovir, lamivudine/emtricitabine, and efavirenz (EFV) in fixed-dose combination tablets. Nevirapine (NVP)-based antiretrovirals (ARVs) are inferior to EFV-based regimens, with poorer viral suppression and increased hepatic and cutaneous side effects. There is some concern about the interaction of RIF and the nonnucleoside analogue reverse-transcriptase inhibitors (NNRTIs) and protease inhibitors (PIs) with increased metabolism via induction of the p-450 cytochrome system. Some suggest increasing the EFV dose when RIF is used, but it is not advised in clinical practice.[14]

■ Differential Diagnosis

Although *M. tuberculosis* is by far the commonest infection in HIV-infected patients, a differential diagnosis must be maintained. Pyogenic causes include the same bacteria as in HIV-negative patient groups, with *Staphylococcus aureus* being the commonest infecting agent, followed by the gram-negative organisms. *Salmonella,* both typhi and nontyphi, may occur. Pyogenic infections tend to cause raised white blood cell (WBC) counts, as opposed to the normal WBC count in *M. tuberculosis*. The imaging is more likely to demonstrate a primary diskitis rather than an osteomyelitis. Management is usually antibiotic treatment, based on the organism cultured and on consultation with the local infectious diseases team. Co-infection of *M. tuberculosis* and pyogenic bacteria is infrequent but does occur. Thus histology, culture, and PCR must be assessed carefully to avoid a misdiagnosis.

Fungal infections also occur in this immunocompromised group. In my experience, it is very rare, with only a handful of cases over the years; yet they need to be identified. This would include *Blastomycosis, Candidiasis*, and *Cryptococcus* (**Figs. 14.2** and **14.3**). Once the infection

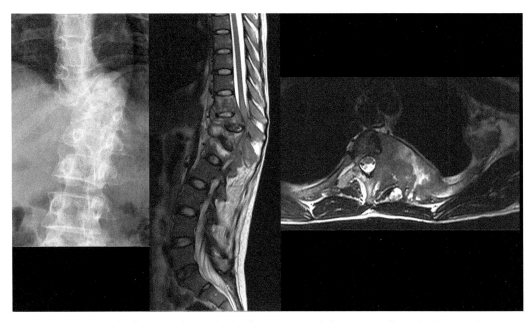

Fig. 14.2 Cryptococcal infection with vertebral collapse and instability. MRI confirms the lung involvement.

is identified, intravenous antifungal treatment should be initiated with conversion to oral agents once a clinical response is observed. A prolonged course of 6 months may be required. Surgery is based on the merits of the case. In the unlikely event that it is diagnosed early in the course of the disease, medical management is all that may be required. More typically,

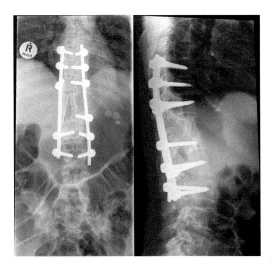

Fig. 14.3 Postoperative views after cryptococcal resection and reconstruction.

there is late presentation or a missed diagnosis and inappropriate initial management, leading to thecal compression and kyphotic collapse. Should the patient's general medical status allow, decompression and reconstruction surgery should be considered. Again, depending on biomechanical requirements, this may be executed either anteriorly or posteriorly, and occasionally both, where the principles of debridement of diseased tissue back to normal bone, biological reconstruction, and instrumented support are followed.

Patients infected with HIV also have an increased incidence of tumor, and this should always be considered. Lymphoma is not uncommonly confused with infection although it tends to involve one vertebral body rather than the disk (as in pyogenic) or two paradiskal vertebrae such as in TB. Biopsy and histological diagnosis is mandatory.

Role of Surgery

Although the mainstay of treatment for spinal TB is medical, surgery may be indicated for ongoing neurologic compromise or predicted

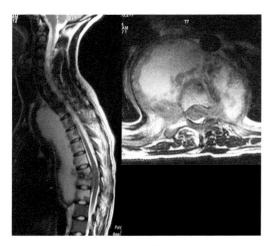

Fig. 14.4 Large paraspinal collection confluent with epidural extension and minimal deformity, ideal for costotransversectomy.

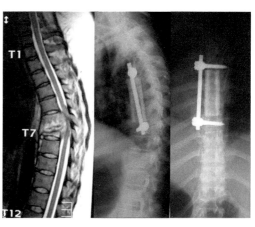

Fig. 14.5 Typical midthoracic spine with tuberculosis (TB), with thecal compression that can be managed with anterior-only debridement, an allograft humerus graft, and simple anterior fixation with pedicle screws into the vertebral body.

or established deformity. In the endemic areas, percutaneous CT-guided biopsies are often not readily available, and the onus of diagnostic biopsy lies with the surgeon. As the biopsy is performed in the operating room, surgeons often include abscess drainage in the procedure to reduce the abscess size, increasing antibiotic penetration and providing symptomatic improvement. This is often the case in large psoas abscesses that would ultimately resorb but cause severe pain, hip flexion deformity, and reduced ambulation due to pain rather than neurologic compromise. A small anterior retroperitoneal approach splitting the external/internal oblique and transversus abdominis fibers enables a minimal approach to achieve this, providing adequate samples for diagnosis and confirmation of drug sensitivity.

As the HIV/TB patient is often in a poor medical condition and unlikely to survive reconstructive surgery, smaller procedures may play a role. In addition, HIV moderates the immune process, often resulting in more abscess formation than bony destruction. Therefore, frequently there is minimal deformity, obviating the need for reconstructive procedures. A costotransversectomy is quick and entails less morbidity, allowing the surgeon not only to obtain samples but also to indirectly decompress the theca, as the abscess is usually confluent with the epidural abscess (**Fig. 14.4**).

In patients with persistent, significant neurologic compromise, especially if the compression is caused by retropulsed osseus-diskal material, decompression and fusion surgery is indicated. Typically, this occurs in the thoracic spine. If midthoracic, a transthoracic decompression and fusion is a good option, allowing direct visualization of the theca. In resource-limited centers, where most of this surgery is performed, humeral allograft provides an inexpensive option with limited instrumentation to prevent dislodgment. Due to the inherent stability provided by the rib cage, little more is required (**Fig. 14.5**). For surgeons who are inexperienced with transthoracic approaches, or in patients who may not survive such invasive surgery, posterior-based vertebral column resection (VCR)-type surgery may be indicated, but far more extensive and expensive instrumentation is required. At the thoracolumbar level, there is far greater inherent biomechanical stress, and anterior-only surgery is likely to fail. Here, anterior and posterior or posterior based VCR-type surgery is indicated (**Fig. 14.6**). In active disease with a flexible deformity, the VCR is far simpler than when it is attempted in rigid deformities.

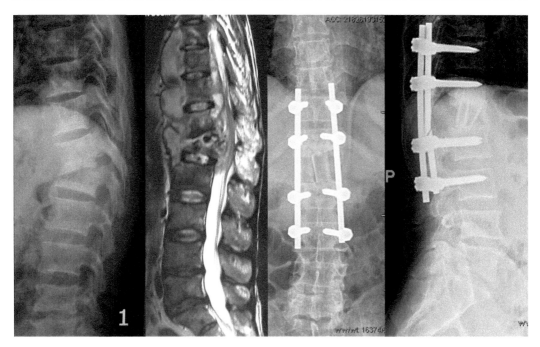

Fig. 14.6 Thoracolumbar TB requiring circumferential decompression and instrumented fusion, all from a posterior approach with a vertebral column resection (VCR) technique.

Deformity correction indications and options are similar to those in HIV-negative patients.

Chapter Summary

Human immunodeficiency virus and tuberculosis drive each other on an immunological basis creating a syndemic in which both diseases coexist. HIV preferentially depletes the *M. tuberculosis*–directed CD4+ cells, reducing the host's defense against *M. tuberculosis* earlier in HIV disease. Thus, *M. tuberculosis* spondylodiskitis is by far the most common cause of spine infection in the HIV-positive cohort.

Tuberculosis presents with vague symptoms in a socioeconomically vulnerable patient group, resulting in delayed presentation, often with advanced disease. Although much less common, a differential diagnosis of pyogenic and fungal infections as well as tumors such as lymphoma needs to be entertained. These entities differ on imaging, with TB typically causing a paraspinal abscess, paradiskal vertebral body destruction, and disk preservation until late in the infection course, whereas pyogenic infections affect the disk first and tumor affects predominantly a single body. However, with HIV co-infection, TB may mimic other conditions with less bone destruction and more pus formation. Intrinsic spinal cord involvement with myelitis may occur without bony involvement.

Biopsy is mandatory with histological examination, culture, and PCR to confirm the diagnosis and determine drug sensitivity.

The mainstay of treatment for spinal TB and other infections is medical, but surgery may be required if there is significant neurological compromise from anterior compression by osseus-diskal debris or predicted or established deformity. Surgery should be tailored to the patients' medical status as they may not tolerate the large insult of reconstructive procedures, and less invasive abscess drainage via costotransversectomy may suffice to drain the abscess and decompress the canal.

Pearls

- In HIV-positive patients presenting with spondylodiskitis, it is tuberculosis until proven otherwise.
- Biopsy is mandatory for establishing the diagnosis by histology, culture, and PCR.
- A prolonged bacterial culture would be helpful because some patients may have TB/bacterial co-infection.
- HIV-positive patients may be in poor general health, necessitating less invasive procedures.

Pitfalls

- Do not treat empirically with antibiotics or anti-TB medications. Preferably confirm the tissue diagnosis and drug sensitivities.
- Do not rely solely on the postoperative ESR to monitor follow-up, as HIV raises the ESR; also monitor weight gain and radiographic healing. Also check for CD4 counts in patients started on antitubercular drugs for fear of initiating IRIS.
- Preferably large-core needles biopsy are required for accurate histological examination.

References

Five Must-Read References

1. World Health Organization. www.who.int/mediacentre/factsheets/fs360/en Accessed February 2016
2. Kwan CK, Ernst JD. HIV and tuberculosis: a deadly human syndemic. Clin Microbiol Rev 2011;24: 351–376
3. World Health Organization. Global Tuberculosis Report, 2016. www.who.org
4. Shankar EM, Vignesh R, Ellegård R, et al. HIV-Mycobacterium tuberculosis co-infection: a "danger-couple model" of disease pathogenesis. Pathog Dis 2014;70:110–118
5. Pawlowski A, Jansson M, Sköld M, Rottenberg ME, Källenius G. Tuberculosis and HIV co-infection. PLoS Pathog 2012;8:e1002464
6. Simon V, Ho DD, Abdool Karim Q. HIV/AIDS epidemiology, pathogenesis, prevention, and treatment. Lancet 2006;368:489–504
7. Rubaihayo J, Tumwesigye NM, Konde-Lule J, Wamani H, Nakku-Joloba E, Makumbi F. Frequency and distribution patterns of opportunistic infections associated with HIV/AIDS in Uganda. BMC Res Notes 2016;9:501
8. Reddy SG, Ali SY, Khalidi A. Study of infections among human immunodeficiency virus/acquired immunodeficiency syndrome patients in Shadan Hospital, Telangana, India. Indian J Sex Transm Dis 2016;37: 147–150
9. Montales M, Chaudhury A, Beebe A. HIV-associated TB syndemic: a growing clinical challenge worldwide. Front Public Health 2015;3:281
10. Weinstein MA, Eismont FJ. Infections of the spine in patients with human immunodeficiency virus. J Bone Joint Surg Am 2005;87:604–609
11. Anley C, Brandt A, Dunn RN. MRI findings of spinal tuberculosis: a comparison of HIV positive and negative patients. Indian J Orthop 2012;46:186–190
12. Polley P, Dunn RN. Non-contiguous spinal tuberculosis: incidence and management. Eur Spinal J 2009;18:1096–1101
13. Held M, Laubscher M, Zar HJ, Dunn RN, Dunn R. GeneXpert polymerase chain reaction for spinal tuberculosis: an accurate and rapid diagnostic test. Bone Joint J 2014;96-B:1366–1369
14. Wasserman S, Meintjes G. The diagnosis, management and prevention of HIV-associated tuberculosis. S Afr Med J 2014;104:886–893

15

Postoperative Spondylodiskitis

Mayan Lendner, Jeffrey Green, Kris E. Radcliff, Joseph S. Butler, Hamadi Murphy, and Alexander R. Vaccaro

Introduction

Postoperative spondylodiskitis (POSD) is an uncommon, yet significant postoperative complication. Spondylodiskitis is a bacterial infection affecting the intervertebral disk space, surrounding bony structures, or soft tissues.[1] Patients with POSD commonly present postoperatively with intense back pain and fever. Most cases occur following surgical procedures in the lumbar region, but also to a lesser extent in the cervical and thoracic regions.[1-4] A recent estimate of the incidence of POSD is 0.21 to 3.6% across all vertebral surgical procedures.[5] Although surgical site infections can occur after spine surgery, spondylodiskitis is a rare complication. Importantly, most spine surgical site infections do not lead to the development of spondylodiskitis. Of course, each spine procedure entails specific and often unique risks.[6] This chapter discusses postoperative spine infections, and specifically postoperative spondylodiskitis. The significance of postoperative infections, the risk factors associated with them, and the current diagnostic, treatment, and prevention strategies are discussed.

General Risk Factors for Spine Infection

There are several well-defined risk factors for surgical site infection (SSI) following spine sur-

gery: are older age, obesity (as measured by the body mass index, BMI), diabetes, cardiovascular disease, and smoking.[6,7] Malnourishment, immunosuppression, hypertension, low serum albumin, and low white blood cell count may also contribute to an increased risk of infection.[6,8] The risk factors relating to the surgery include longer operative times and increased levels of surgical invasiveness.[6,9] Long periods of immobilization postoperatively may increase the risk of infection.[8] Specific risk factors for spine SSI include the surgical approach (posterior approaches have a greater risk for infection than anterior approaches), and the length of the incision (longer incisions are associated with a greater incidence of infection).[8] Spine surgery in the setting of trauma is associated with a higher risk of SSI.[8]

However, despite these well-defined risks for SSI, there are no patient or procedural risk factors identified for POSD. We have found that POSD is often a late occurrence following SSI in cases that have been treated in a subacute or delayed manner, although this may not be true in all cases. POSD may also occur in the early postoperative period in patients who are immunosuppressed.

Pathology and Bacteriology

Postoperative spondylodiskitis most often develops in the disk space following intradiskal procedures. Although rare, hematogenous spread can occur from other regions of the body. The specific bacteriology of POSD is largely unknown. We suspect that the most common bacterial causes of SSI are also the common causes of POSD. In one study, biopsy-confirmed infection in the disk space was observed to be caused by a single organism in 51% of patients, by two organisms in 16%, and by more than two organisms in 8%.[10]

Diagnosis

Overview and Complicating Factors in Diagnosis

Postoperative spondylodiskitis is difficult to diagnose due to the indolent nature in which the infection presents and the limitations in diagnostic accuracy of existing investigative strategies.[11] In most cases, postoperative wound infections present with prolonged wound drainage, axial pain, and a variety of red flag symptoms including fevers or chills. Given the common nature of these symptoms in the acute postoperative period, the diagnosis of POSD can be confounded by other conditions.[12] Furthermore, low back pain in postoperative spine patients is generally an expected symptom.[13] Patients with POSD may exhibit atypical, nonmechanical back or neck pain that is worse when the patient is in the supine position and worse at night. This atypical pain is suggestive of an infectious process, as opposed to normal postoperative muscle healing. However, the axial pain from POSD may be initially overlooked because it is confounded by the patient's baseline pain or new axial pain from the procedure.[13]

Imaging

Plain Radiography

The first imaging modality of choice is plain radiographs.[12,14] Unfortunately, most studies agree that the effectiveness of plain radiographs is limited in the early diagnosis of spondylodiskitis due to the lack of end-plate destruction. Disk space narrowing is a late radiographic sign of diskitis. As the infection progresses, destruction of the bony end plates or fractures become more apparent.[12,14]

Magnetic Resonance Imaging

The most frequently used imaging modality for diagnosing POSD is magnetic resonance imaging (MRI).[12–14] MRI illustrates the bone, nerve, disk, ligament, and muscle structures in anatomic detail.[12] MRI is very sensitive for early spondylodiskitis due to the presence of fluid and contrast uptake in the vertebral bodies and end plates.[14] Specific MRI findings in cases of spondylodiskitis include a high disk space and vertebral body T2 signal on short tau inversion recovery (STIR) images, as well as a low disk space and vertebral body T1 signal, and contrast uptake (**Fig. 15.1**). MRI may show the presence of irregular edema and inflammation of the epidural space or an epidural abscess.[13] Nonetheless, MRI is not without its limitations. Bone edema on MRI can be caused by other, noninfectious sources, such as a fracture, spinal osteotomy, or spinal instrumentation. MRI is also susceptible to metallic artifact, so the resolution around instrumentation is often suboptimal.[15] Finally, MRI is highly sensitive but not specific. Thus, normal postoperative epidural fluid collection observed in MRI can be confused with POSD. Pathology identified on MRI of the spinal column may be indicative of other preexisting pathology (i.e., aging, degeneration from overuse, past traumatic injury) and not specifically spondylodiskitis.[13,14] Unfortunately, a recent study found that routine use of MRI may not be effective in monitoring the natural history of effectively treated osteodiskitis due to the lack of pertinent clinical correlation.[14]

Computed Tomography

Computed tomography (CT) has demonstrated less specificity and sensitivity compared with MRI in the diagnosis of POSD.[12] Despite the increased preference for MRI, CT scans still hold some value in the diagnosis and treatment of spondylodiskitis. Bone involvement is a hallmark feature of osteodiskitis. CT scans (especially three-dimensional CT) can give a

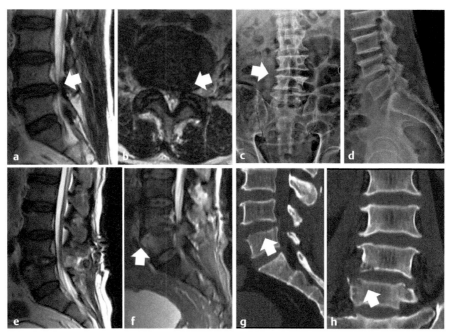

Fig. 15.1 A 54-year-old man presents with post-operative diskitis. **(a,b)** Imaging demonstrates left lower limb radiculopathy due to diskogenic stenosis *(arrow)*. Due to unrelenting radicular pain, the patient underwent microdecompression and diskectomy. During the third postoperative week, he presented with significant back pain and recurrence of leg pain. He had significantly walking disability and walked with a list. **(c,d)** Plain radiographs showed only a mild sciatic scoliosis toward the right side *(arrow)*. **(e,f)** T2 and short tau inversion recovery (STIR) sagittal magnetic resonance imaging (MRI) sequences show the typical findings of diskitis: hyperintense fluid signal in the disk space, subchondral marrow edema, and irregular end plates *(arrow)*. **(g,h)** Computed tomography (CT) scan findings were unremarkable except for subtle subchondral lucencies and asymmetric collapse of the disk space *(arrow)*. Because there was no gross instability, the patient was treated with debridement and antibiotics.

more complete picture of the degree of bony destruction.[12,14]

Nuclear Scintigraphy

Nuclear scintigraphy imaging (NSI) involves the injection of radioactive isotopes. Nuclear medicine studies are generally not sensitive in the axial skeleton.[11] However, new advances in NSI may lead to decreased infection detection times and higher sensitivity.[14] One radioactive agent that has seen success is gallium 67, which is more preferentially taken up by areas of infection.[14]

Emerging Imaging Modalities: ^{18}F-FDG-PET

[18]F-fluorodeoxyglucose (FDG)–positron emission tomography (PET) is a variant of nuclear scintigraphy in which gamma rays emitted by a positron tracer are captured. It may offer significant potential as an imaging modality for detecting spondylodiskitis, perhaps with even greater sensitivity and specificity than MRI.[12,14] Results of ^{18}F-FDG-PET testing are often available within 2 hours of tracer injection and the study is not affected by the presence of metallic artifact (i.e., from medical implants).[14] ^{18}F-FDG normally demonstrates minimal uptake in

Table 15.1 Standard Erythrocyte Sedimentation Rate (ESR), C-Reactive Protein (CRP), and Procalcitonin (PCT) Levels Following Surgery (Without Infection)[18,19]

	Half-Life	Detectable	Peak	Normalize
ESR	Fibrinogen: 100 hours; immunoglobulin G > 1 week	24 hours	> 1 week	Several weeks
CRP	18 hours	6–12 hours	24–48 hours	1 week
PCT	24–35 hours	2–4 hours	12–24 hours	1–2 days

bone marrow, and therefore changes consistent with infection are likely to increase tracer uptake and highlight a specific region on the scan.[12] ^{18}F-FDG-PET is also capable of assisting in the differentiation between degenerative disease and infection when used in combination with MRI.[14] One currently observed drawback is that it may fail to differentiate between malignant tumors and infection due to similar uptake of the tracer.[12,14]

Laboratory Measurements

Blood tests and cultures are regarded as effective tools in the diagnosis of spondylodiskitis.[12] Biopsy is indicated if the organism is unknown, such as if blood cultures are negative. CT-guided needle aspiration for biopsy has been used with mixed results.[16] One study with a small sample size demonstrated an associated diagnostic accuracy of 50%.[12] Larger tissue samples recovered at the time of surgical exploration are more accurate when testing for infection, but are associated with the complications of a more invasive procedure, and the accuracy is only 75%.[12] In addition to blood cultures, standard laboratory tests include complete blood count (CBC), erythrocyte sedimentation rate (ESR), and C-reactive protein.[14] However, many of these markers remain elevated for many weeks postoperatively.[14] CRP and serum amyloid A (SAA) have been investigated as more specific infection biomarkers, as their levels usually peak within 3 days, potentially before the clinical presentation of infection.[14] SAA may offer several advantages over CRP, in that it has a shorter half-life and thus a shorter time to return to preoperative baseline values. Moreover, SAA has also been shown to be gender and age

neutral and, unlike CRP, not affected in the presence of corticosteroids exposure. Given the immense potential for confusion surrounding these laboratory exams, it would be beneficial to have established baseline values preoperatively to monitor laboratory values periodically in patients suspected of developing a postoperative spinal infection. Another marker that may be considered as an indicator of infection is procalcitonin (PCT), although current research has provided mixed results.[17] In our experience, PCT level is both a sensitive and specific serum marker of infection. PCT is superior to CRP in differentiating infection from other sources of inflammation such as normal postsurgery inflammation.[18] Due to the short half-life, the change in PCT is responsive to treatment (**Table 15.1**). One study, however, demonstrated that PCT elevation was not useful in differentiating patients with spondylodiskitis from those with a disk herniation.[14]

◾ Specific Prevention of Infection

Surgical Time

Prolonged surgical time can affect the colonization of implants, surgical tools, and incision sites.[20] Implant contamination risk will increase over time regardless of precautions, but simply covering the implant set reduces contamination rates significantly as compared with uncovered sets.[21,22] Preincision in-room time or anesthesia ready time (ART) greater than 1 hour has been shown to significantly increase the infection risk, with August and September being the months most likely to have ARTs greater than 1 hour.[20,23]

Topical Vancomycin Powder

Another form of infection prevention that is now in favor is topical vancomycin powder (TVP). Numerous studies have shown its effectiveness in reducing the infection rate as compared with historical treatments, with no decrease in the rates of fusion or increase in renal toxicity.[24,25] Topical vancomycin has also proven to be cost-effective.[26] Despite positive research on the effectiveness of TVP, several studies suggest that TVP has no effect on infection rates at all and is no more effective than standard alcohol foam in infection prevention.[27,28] Some studies also suggest that TVP may increase the rate of gram-negative infection.[29]

Treatment of Infection

Several scoring systems have been developed to help physicians decide which treatment is best suited for which patient. The Spondylodiskitis Severity Code developed by Homagk et al,[1] classifies patients with POSD into three grades of severity based on their clinical and laboratory parameters, the degree of morphological vertebral destruction as seen on radiological examinations, and neurological status. Therapies ranging from antibiotic treatment to specific surgical interventions can then be applied based on the patients' severity grade.

Conservative Nonsurgical Treatment

Although some studies suggest that the duration of antibiotic treatment and the number of surgical debridements have no effect on remission rates in POSD, antibiotic therapy remains the standard of care to treat infections of all kinds.[30] A treatment regimen of > 12 weeks is recommended, as it is associated with recurrence rates below 5%.[30] Generally, therapy is withheld until culture and sensitivity testing

is completed. Selecting the appropriate antibiotic should be guided by the pathogen identified; however, broad-spectrum antibiotics covering the most commonly associated pathogens may be used when a biopsy is unavailable.[31] In the case of sepsis, there may be no time to perform a biopsy as urgent antimicrobial therapy is indicated. Initial parenteral treatment is preferred, usually lasting 3 to 8 weeks followed by oral treatment for up to 1 year.[10] Positive blood cultures and neurologic abnormalities usually indicate the need for a longer parenteral course.[10] Discontinuation of therapy is indicated when the selected duration of antibiotic exposure is ended, the symptoms resolve, and ESR and CRP values normalize.[10] A weekly reduction of CRP level by 50% is indicative of successful treatment.[10] A spinal orthosis can be used to prevent deformity and manage pain while the patient is on antibiotics.

Surgical Treatment

When medical management remains ineffective, or instability develops, or kyphosis, scoliosis, progressive neurologic deficit, sepsis, extensive bony destruction, epidural abscess, or intractable pain presents as a result of POSD, then surgery may be required.[31–37]

Surgery and Approach

Surgery is an effective form of treatment for POSD. Surgery is the first line of treatment in the setting of sepsis, epidural abscess formation, or progressive neurologic deficit. Surgery should be considered in cases that have failed medical management and are progressing with subsequent osteomyelitis. Surgery is also of benefit in the presence of postinfectious instability and progressive deformity.

The surgical approach depends mainly on the patient's clinical presentation. A debridement is recommended if there is an acute neurological deficit with no evidence of instability. Posterior debridement (usually a laminoforaminotomy or laminectomy) enables a rapid decompression of patients with cauda equina syndrome or septicemia who are too unstable for a longer reconstructive procedure.

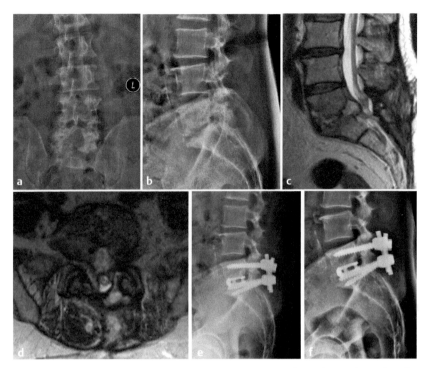

Fig. 15.2 A 53-year-old patient presents after having undergone L5-S1 diskectomy at another hospital. He was asymptomatic for 1 month and then developed gradual-onset back pain and radiculopathy. He had undergone debridement by the primary surgeon but his infection persisted. When he presented to us, he was bed-bound, with significant disability and mild sepsis. **(a,b)** Radiographs and **(c,d)** MRI showed a frank diskitis and epidural abscess at L5-S1. **(e)** Because there was recurrent and persistent infection, he was treated with debridement and instrumented fusion, and prolonged antibiotic therapy. **(f)** Follow-up radiograph performed at 6 months shows good healing of the lesion.

Additionally, an initial debridement may be performed in patients who are acutely bacteremic or have copious purulent material. Endoscopic debridement is an elegant way to obtain an open biopsy or to treat patients who are medically unable to undergo a decompressive surgery. We do not have significant experience in the utilization of endoscopic debridement to treat patients with neurologic deficit.

Arthrodesis is indicated in the setting of POSD when there is instability or potential instability (such as a pathological fracture, deformity, or spondylolisthesis). Instrumentation is commonly used in spine fusions even in the setting of active infection (**Fig. 15.2**). In some cases, percutaneous instrumentation may reduce the risk of wound complications associated with open instrumentation when stabilization is necessary. Autograft is the ideal bone graft.

Allograft can become colonized by infected material, as it is nonvital tissue. There is some concern that artificial surfaces, such as polyetheretherketone (PEEK), can become colonized by bacteria. Titanium has a natural passivation/oxidation that renders it less susceptible to long-term colonization. Our practice is to use an autograft when possible, but, if necessary, titanium cages can be used to treat cavitary defects. However, such cavitary defects are rare in the treatment of spondylodiskitis.

◾ Chapter Summary

Postoperative spondylodiskitis is a rare yet significant type of postoperative spine infection. Occurring most commonly in the lumbar region, POSD involves infection of the intervertebral disk and surrounding tissue. With the ever-increasing prevalence of invasive surgical procedures, surgeons must become more informed of the risk factors and significance of POSD as well as the most up-to-date methods of prevention, diagnosis, and treatment. With symptoms common to most postoperative spine patients, POSD can be difficult to diagnose early. Radiological and laboratory findings help clinicians make more timely diagnoses of POSD if such a process is suspected. Although recent studies suggest newer imaging modalities such as ^{18}F-FDG-PET may prove useful, MRI still remains the most studied and effective imaging modality for diagnosis. Blood cultures are useful, but CRP, procalcitonin, and SAA have gained favor as the most predictive serum markers for diagnosis. Prevention is the first step in the treatment of POSD; surgeons must take precautions to avoid lengthy operative times and should avoid practices that may potentially compromise the sterility of implants in the operating room. Topical vancomycin powder has gained favor due to its cost-effectiveness and its clinical effectiveness. Antibiotics remain the most effective nonsurgical treatment for infection. Although *Staphylococcus aureus* remains the most common causative pathogen of POSD, other, rarer organisms such as *Propionibacterium Acnes* must be considered. In cases of sepsis, epidural abscess formation, and progressive neurologic deficit, surgery is the first line of treatment along with antibiotics. The anterior approach is the preferred surgical approach when both the vertebral body and disk space are involved. It is important that health care providers understand and be prepared for the potential complication of POSD in all spine surgery patients.

Pearls

- Age, obesity, diabetes, cardiovascular disease, and smoking are all significant risk factors for the development of postoperative spondylodiskitis, but the invasiveness of many spine surgeries and the prolonged operating time increase this risk further.
- *Staphylococcus aureus* is the most common form of bacterial infection found in cases of spondylodiskitis.
- Repeat laboratory testing along with MRI are currently the most successful approaches in diagnosing postoperative spondylodiskitis.
- Decreasing the procedure time and the anesthesia ready time, an increased focus on sterility, and the use of topical vancomycin powder have all been shown to be effective in reducing the incidence of postoperative spinal infections.
- A long course of antibiotics, prescribing, when possible, the most target-specific drugs, remains the best approach for the treatment of postoperative spondylodiskitis. Surgery is also an effective treatment method in cases that prove to be resistant to nonoperative care.

Pitfalls

- Do not overlook the complaints of severe disproportionate lower back pain in postoperative patients, as it may be an indicator of early postoperative spondylodiskitis.
- Do not rely solely on laboratory and imaging results, as they can be altered in both the infected and noninfected patient postoperatively.

References
Five Must-Read References

1. Homagk L, Homagk N, Klauss JR, Roehl K, Hofmann GO, Marmelstein D. Spondylodiscitis severity code: scoring system for the classification and treatment of non-specific spondylodiscitis. Eur Spine J 2016;25: 1012–1020
2. Espitalier F, de Keating-Hart A, Morinière S, et al. Cervical spondylodiscitis following an invasive procedure on the neopharynx after circumferential pharyngolaryngectomy: a retrospective case series. Eur Spine J 2016;25:3894–3901
3. González-Paz T, Nehme-Paz AR, Rodríguez-Acevedo N, Arán-González I. Espondilodiscitis cervical secundaria a inserción de prótesis fonatoria. Acta Otorrinolaringol Esp 2016;67:239–241
4. Hahn BS, Kim K-H, Kuh S-U, et al. Surgical treatment in patients with cervical osteomyelitis: single

institute's experiences. Korean J Spine 2014;11:162–168

5. Pourbagher A, Tok S, Aslan H. Laboratuvar Testleri Pozitif Olmadan Magnetik Rezonans Görüntüleme ile Tanı Konulan Postoperatif Spondilodiskitis ve Epidural Abse. Cukurova Medical Journal 2015;40:97

6. Parchi PD, Evangelisti G, Andreani L, et al. Postoperative spine infections. Orthop Rev (Pavia) 2015;7:5900

7. Maruo K, Berven SH. Outcome and treatment of postoperative spine surgical site infections: predictors of treatment success and failure. J Orthop Sci 2014;19:398–404

8. Saeedinia S, Nouri M, Azarhomayoun A, et al. The incidence and risk factors for surgical site infection after clean spinal operations: a prospective cohort study and review of the literature. Surg Neurol Int 2015;6:154

9. Tominaga H, Setoguchi T, Ishidou Y, Nagano S, Yamamoto T, Komiya S. Risk factors for surgical site infection and urinary tract infection after spine surgery. Eur Spine J 2016;25:3908–3915

10. Gouliouris T, Aliyu SH, Brown NM. Spondylodiscitis: update on diagnosis and management. J Antimicrob Chemother 2010;65(Suppl 3):iii11–iii24

11. Termaat MF, Raijmakers PGHM, Scholten HJ, Bakker FC, Patka P, Haarman HJTM. The accuracy of diagnostic imaging for the assessment of chronic osteomyelitis: a systematic review and meta-analysis. J Bone Joint Surg Am 2005;87:2464–2471

12. Sobottke R, Seifert H, Fätkenheuer G, Schmidt M, Gossmann A, Eysel P. Current diagnosis and treatment of spondylodiscitis. Dtsch Arztebl Int 2008;105:181–187

13. Kaliaperumal C, Kuechler D, Kaar G, Marks C, O'Sullivan M. Does surgical technique affect the incidence of spondylodiscitis post-lumbar microdiscectomy? A retrospective analysis of 3063 patients. Spine 2013;38:364–367

14. Chahoud J, Kanafani Z, Kanj SS. Surgical site infections following spine surgery: eliminating the controversies in the diagnosis. Front Med (Lausanne) 2014;1:7

15. Kimura H, Shikata J, Odate S, Soeda T. Pedicle screw fluid sign: an indication on magnetic resonance imaging of a deep infection after posterior spinal instrumentation. Clin Spine Surg 2017;30:169–175

16. Jo JE, Miller AO, Cohn MR, Nemani VM, Schneider R, Lebl DR. Evaluating the diagnostic yield of computed tomography-guided aspirations in suspected post-operative spine infections. HSS J 2016;12:119–124

17. Faqi MK, Al-Qahtani M, Elmusharaf K. The roles of procalcitonin, C-reactive protein and erythrocyte sedimentation rate in predicting bacteremia. J Immunol Infect Dis [Internet] 2015;2

18. Chung YG, Won YS, Kwon YJ, Shin HC, Choi CS, Yeom J-S. Comparison of serum CRP and procalcitonin in patients after spine surgery. J Korean Neurosurg Soc 2011;49:43–48

19. Mayo Medical Laboratories. 2018 https://www.mayomedicallaboratories.com/index.html

20. Puffer RC, Murphy M, Maloney P, et al. Increased total anesthetic time leads to higher rates of surgical site infections in spinal fusions. Spine 2017;42:E687–E690

21. Menekse G, Kuscu F, Suntur BM, et al. Evaluation of the time-dependent contamination of spinal implants: prospective randomized trial. Spine 2015;40:1247–1251

22. Litrico S, Recanati G, Gennari A, Maillot C, Saffarini M, Le Huec J-C. Single-use instrumentation in posterior lumbar fusion could decrease incidence of surgical site infection: a prospective bi-centric study. Eur J Orthop Surg Traumatol 2016;26:21–26

23. Radcliff KE, Rasouli MR, Neusner A, et al. Preoperative delay of more than 1 hour increases the risk of surgical site infection. Spine 2013;38:1318–1323

24. Pahys JM, Pahys JR, Cho SK, et al. Methods to decrease postoperative infections following posterior cervical spine surgery. J Bone Joint Surg Am 2013;95:549–554

25. Armaghani SJ, Menge TJ, Lovejoy SA, Mencio GA, Martus JE. Safety of topical vancomycin for pediatric spinal deformity: nontoxic serum levels with supratherapeutic drain levels. Spine 2014;39:1683–1687

26. Theologis AA, Demirkiran G, Callahan M, Pekmezci M, Ames C, Deviren V. Local intrawound vancomycin powder decreases the risk of surgical site infections in complex adult deformity reconstruction: a cost analysis. Spine 2014;39:1875–1880

27. Martin JR, Adogwa O, Brown CR, et al. Experience with intrawound vancomycin powder for posterior cervical fusion surgery. J Neurosurg Spine 2015;22:26–33

28. Tubaki VR, Rajasekaran S, Shetty AP. Effects of using intravenous antibiotic only versus local intrawound vancomycin antibiotic powder application in addition to intravenous antibiotics on postoperative infection in spine surgery in 907 patients. Spine 2013;38:2149–2155

29. Ghobrial GM, Thakkar V, Andrews E, et al. Intraoperative vancomycin use in spinal surgery: single institution experience and microbial trends. Spine 2014;39:550–555

30. Billières J, Uçkay I, Faundez A, et al. Variables associated with remission in spinal surgical site infections. J Spine Surg 2016;2:128–134

31. Cornett CA, Vincent SA, Crow J, Hewlett A. Bacterial spine infections in adults: evaluation and management. J Am Acad Orthop Surg 2016;24:11–18

32. Lall RR, Wong AP, Lall RR, Lawton CD, Smith ZA, Dahdaleh NS. Evidence-based management of deep wound infection after spinal instrumentation. J Clin Neurosci 2015;22:238–242

33. Lee JS, Ahn DK, Chang BK, Lee JI. Treatment of surgical site infection in posterior lumbar interbody fusion. Asian Spine J 2015;9:841–848

34. Dipaola CP, Saravanja DD, Boriani L, et al. Postoperative infection treatment score for the spine (PITSS): construction and validation of a predictive model to define need for single versus multiple irrigation and debridement for spinal surgical site infection. Spine J 2012;12:218–230

35. Ousey KJ, Atkinson RA, Williamson JB, Lui S. Negative pressure wound therapy (NPWT) for spinal wounds: a systematic review. Spine J 2013;13:1393–1405

36. Zwolak P, König MA, Osterhoff G, Wilzeck V, Simmen H-P, Jukema GN. Therapy of acute and delayed spinal infections after spinal surgery treated with negative pressure wound therapy in adult patients. Orthop Rev (Pavia) 2013;5:e30

37. Rohmiller MT, Akbarnia BA, Raiszadeh K, Raiszadeh K, Canale S. Closed suction irrigation for the treatment of postoperative wound infections following posterior spinal fusion and instrumentation. Spine 2010;35:642–646

16

Postoperative Peri-Implant Spine Infections

Claudio Lamartina, Alex Vesnaver, and Carlotta Martini

◼ Introduction

Postoperative spinal infections are one of the most troublesome complications. Despite advances in drug development, innovation of surgical technique, and postoperative care, wound infection is still one of the major threats in spine surgery.[1] Postoperative spinal infections are responsible for significant morbidity and mortality,[2] and are related to adverse postoperative events such as nonunion, neurologic sequelae, chronic pain, and deformity. The National Nosocomial Infections Surveillance Summary System of the Centers for Disease Control and Prevention (CDC) recently reported rates of surgical site infection (SSI) in spine surgery ranging from 0 to 20%, based on different definitions of infection.[3] These fluctuations depend on the indications for surgery, the anatomic site, the approach, the presence of instrumentation, the type of infection, and the extent of the infection.[1] Moreover, SSIs are multifactorial, and risk factors include microbial-related, patient-related, and procedure-related factors. From a financial perspective, postoperative infections in spine surgery are responsible for at least a two-fold increase in health-related and social costs. Readmission and reoperation rates have been estimated to be around 65% in a recent publication from the Surgical Infection Society.[2]

An established risk factor for postoperative infection in spine surgery is the use of implants.[4] This chapter discusses the best evidence-based measures that should be adopted to identify, correctly manage, and finally minimize infection rates in instrumented spine surgery.

Some guidelines are available for antibiotic prophylaxis[5] and for antisepsis.[6] But some questions have not been adequately addressed in the literature, such as the following:

- Is surgical debridement always required, and when?
- When is removal of instrumentation required?
- What is the ideal postoperative care and monitoring for postoperative peri-implant infection patients?
- What are the main risk factors for postoperative infections?

We address these issues as well as the best evidence available in the literature. We also discuss a complex case from our practice.

◼ Diagnosis

Early Postoperative Infection

Postoperative peri-implant infections can present in a very clear, evident way or in a more subtle, hidden setting. According to the CDC standard definition of SSI, all the peri-implant infections are "organ/space" infections[7] because they usually extend beyond the underlying fascia and muscle layers, with the involvement of the posterior bony elements of the vertebrae, of the zygapophyseal joints, and sometimes suspicion of the intervertebral disk. The clinical suspect of peri-implant infection can arise from one or more of the following observations:

- Persistent pain at the surgical incision
- Fluid collection under the wound, with or without purulent drainage
- Slow wound healing

Among these, pain is the most frequent clinical finding,[8] with a reported prevalence of almost 100%. Fever is not a significant sign for peri-implant infection.

The most frequent causative organism is *Staphylococcus aureus* (85%), and among these patients, there is a significant percentage of methicillin-resistant bacteria (30%), especially after revision surgery. Gram-negative organisms are less frequently involved. Presumably infection from gram-negative agents can be related to surgery in the lower lumbar spine and sacroiliac area.

Diagnostic workup of peri-implant infection involves laboratory investigations and imaging studies.

The white blood cell count is an unreliable indicator of infection, because altered levels could be the effect of drugs (e.g., corticosteroids) or hemodilution, for example. The acute-phase reactants C-reactive protein (CRP) and erythrocyte sedimentation rate (ESR) are more useful for diagnosing infection but must be interpreted with respect to the time since the index surgery. ESR remains altered for up to 6 weeks after surgery, whereas CRP levels normalize within 2 weeks. Hence, abnormal CRP levels in the follow-up of a spinal instrumented surgical procedure should always be monitored and investigated,[8] and CRP is considered the more sensitive indicator of the presence of SSI.

As a consequence, imaging is usually performed to get a deeper insight, and in the vast majority of cases magnetic resonance imaging (MRI) is the first choice. Contrast-enhancement improves MRI accuracy in detecting infection. Interpretation should take into account the time from index surgery, because tissue disruption and subsequent edema and blood collection could mimic infection-related signs.

In patients with absolute contraindications for MRI, a computed tomography (CT) scan is the best option. Radiographs are not as useful as MRI or CT scan, but in some cases of delayed or chronic infections they can be informative. The presence of radiolucency around the screws, bone erosion, end-plate disruption, or implant pullout in the absence of any mechanical major issue or together with clinical features can be highly suggestive of peri-implant infection.

Delayed Postoperative Infections

Ninety percent of infections occur early in the postoperative period. Only 10% are delayed; that is, they occur 3 months or longer after surgery.[9] There are two main pathogenetic hypotheses for this delay:

1. Atypical agents and uncommon pathogens spawn the infection slowly and insidiously, making the diagnosis difficult and delaying it. The infection may sometimes be taking place since the early postoperative period but remains unrecognized. The most frequently responsible agent is *Propionibacterium acnes*.[10]
2. The implant is colonized by hematogenous seeding, resulting from a distant invasive procedure with transient bacteriemia (dental surgery, gastroenteric, or urinary endoscopy).

There is scientific evidence of hematogenous infection in hip and knee arthroplasty.[11] The consensus guideline of the American Academy of Orthopaedic Surgeons strongly recommends performing antibiotic prophylaxis before any invasive medical procedure for patients with total joint prosthetic implants.[12] Conversely, no guidelines are available for similar procedures in patients with spinal implants.

Table 16.1 The Mean Time Interval from Surgery and Infection Onset in Infections Caused by Different Bacterial Types

Organism	Days from Index Surgery
Staphylococcus aureus	19
Staphylococcus epidermidis	22
Enterobacter spp.	23
Propionibacterium spp.	37
Gram-negative	15

Source: Adapted from Abdul-Jabbar A, Takemoto S, Weber MH, et al. Surgical site infection in spinal surgery: description of surgical and patient-based risk factors for postoperative infection using administrative claims data. Spine 2012;37:1340–1345.

Lewkonia and colleagues[13] retrospectively reviewed patients with delayed perioperative infections, and sought a possible cause–effect relationship between invasive medical procedures and infection. At the same time, they submitted a survey to a group of selected, expert spine surgeons, asking about the administration of antibiotic prophylaxis for an invasive medical procedure in patients with spinal implants. With all the limitations due to the retrospective nature of the study, it seems unlikely that hematogenous seeding would be responsible for delayed infection. This is in line with the experts' advising against the prophylaxis in spinal patients before invasive medical procedures.

Interestingly, it has been shown that delayed infections are closely related to scoliosis surgery, but not with the number of fused levels. This could be related to such features of scoliosis surgery as the need for blood transfusion and the use of bone allograft, for example.[14] Moreover, delayed peri-implant infections are frequently culture-negative. The typical bacteriological profile of them, in fact, is made up of less virulent pathogens.

Table 16.1 shows the time to onset of infection from the index surgery in postoperative spine infections.

◼ Treatment

Debridement

When a peri-implant infection is diagnosed, immediate washout and surgical debridement with intraoperative sampling should be performed.[15,16] The use of drains is supported by our personal experience and by the available literature. Some surgeons routinely use continuous irrigation to avoid repetitive surgical debridement,[17] but in our experience a single washout procedure has been shown to be effective for nearly all the early peri-implant postoperative infections. The advantages of this quick, simple procedure are as follows:

- It provides the microbiological information necessary to correctly target the antibiotic therapy. Intraoperative samples are the gold standard for the laboratory identification of pathogens.
- The removal of purulent material and necrotic avascular tissue facilitates drug delivery and eradication of infective foci.
- The placement of a drain facilitates wound closure and healing, and reduces the fluid collection and the subsequent bacterial regrowth.

Evidence-based data support the improved outcome when surgical washout and debridement for early infections are performed immediately after an infection diagnosis.[18]

For delayed infections, the same procedure has shown lower efficacy, and there is a slight need for implant removal. This is probably related to the presence of a structured, resistant biofilm.

Thus, the answer to the question about when to perform surgical debridement in cases of diagnosed postoperative peri-implant spinal infection is as soon as the diagnosis is made. The success rate is high for early (within 1 month from index surgery) postoperative infections, but even in delayed infections, it is important to obtain intraoperative samples to correctly address pathogens.

Implant Retention/Removal

It is debated whether implant retention or removal would be the better solution for postoperative peri-implant infections. There are important differences between early and delayed peri-implant infections management.

Early

The available literature favors retention of implants in early infection.[16,18–21] Some interesting data recently reported by Kanayama and colleagues[22] provide initial evidence that in cases with clear osteomyelitis or vertebral abscess, implant removal is mandatory from the very beginning. These authors, in their retrospective review on 1,445 patients, found that patients with peri-implant infection with a positive MRI for the aforementioned findings were more likely to undergo repetitive failed surgeries, with progressive bone destruction and a nonunion rate of 75%. Removing the hardware seems to be the most appropriate step for these patients, and the authors feel that it should probably have been adopted from the first surgical revision procedure. Implant exchange is a suitable option in this situation, in cases of a severe clinical presentation (i.e., acute sepsis) after a careful evaluation of the risk-benefit balance for the patient, especially in deformity correction or severe postsurgical instability (i.e., three-column osteotomies). Interbody devices are usually left in place. The need for removal of an interbody device is usually a consequence of antibiotic therapy failure, because the risk-benefit profile is, in cases of early infections, against the revision of the interbody device.

In our experience, we have successfully retained instrumentation in all the early peri-implant postoperative infections.

Delayed

The general consensus in the literature is that implants should be removed in cases of delayed infections.[20,23–25] Attempts at hardware retention lead to high infection recurrence rates. With hardware removal, successful eradication of infection is more likely to be achieved. In the majority of cases, the infection is responsible for nonunion, so implant removal is related to an increased risk of progressive deformity, with the need of further corrective surgery. This potential complication should always be considered, and patients should be informed about the possible need for a reoperation for a deformity correction in the future.

A recent retrospective case-control study by Tominaga and colleagues[26] focused on the risk factors related to unavoidable hardware removal. They found that revision surgery with multiple previous procedures, low preoperative hemoglobin (Hb) values, high preoperative serum creatinine values, and the presence of methicillin-resistant *Staphylococcus aureus* are statistically related to hardware removal. Another parameter known as the postoperative infection treatment score for the spine (PITSS) has been found to be related to implant removal. This scoring system tries to identify those patients at risk for multiple, repeated surgical washout and debridement procedures. The predictive model has been validated over a 4-year period, and the results have been published by DiPaola et al.[27] The scoring system in summarized in **Table 16.2**. A score between 7 and 14 is defined as low risk for repeated surgical debridement; between 15 and 20 is defined as undetermined risk; 21 or above is high risk, which correlates with the likelihood of hardware removal. Patients with clearly unstable segments but with a likelihood of hardware removal can be selected for hardware exchange, as follows:

1. Remove the existing colonized implants with their biofilm.
2. Preserve neurologic function, preventing injuries secondary to instability.

This is a halfway choice in cases of delayed infections, but to be seriously considered when the neurologic risks of hardware removal are high.

An interbody device in late infections should be managed similarly. After removal of the colonized device, infected tissues can be harvested and a bone graft or trabecular tantalum cage should be used.

Table 16.2 Postoperative Infection Treatment Score for the Spine (PITSS) Scoring System

Predictor	PITSS Score
Spine location	
Cervical	1
Thoracolumbar	2
Lumbosacral	4
Comorbidities	
None/other	0
Cardiovascular/pulmonary	1
Diabetes	4
Microbiology	
Gram-positive	2
Gram-negative or polymicrobial without MRSA	4
MRSA (alone or poly)	6
Distant site infection	
None	1
Urinary/pneumonia	3
Bacteriemia alone	5
Bacteriemia + PNA/UTI	6
Instrumentation	
Yes	6
No	2
Bone graft	
None	1
Autograft	3
Other (allograft, BMP, synthetic)	6

Abbreviations: BMP, bone morphogenetic protein; MRSA, methicillin-resistant *Staphylococcus aureus*; PNA, pneumonia; UTI, urinary tract infection.
Source: DiPaola CP, Saravanja DD, Boriani L, et al. Postoperative infection treatment score for the spine (PITSS): construction and validation of a predictive model to define need for single versus multiple irrigation and debridement for spinal surgical site infection. Spine J 2012;12:218–230.

In our experience the only patient who has been selected for implant removal was a paraplegic teenager, whose case follows.

▪ Case Study

G.C. is a 24-year-old man with a history of traumatic spinal cord injury sustained in a motor vehicle accident that occurred in 2010. The thoracic fracture is a T7-T8 type C N4 according to the new AOSpine traumatic fracture classification. Concomitant splenic and pancreatic rupture and pulmonary insufficiency due to multiple contusions secondary to the trauma were observed and treated. The first surgical spinal procedure was a posterior T6–T12 fixation. No recovery from the neurologic deficit was observed after surgery, and the patient has been paraplegic since then, with a mid-thoracic sensorimotor level, with deep sensory perception intact. After 4 months the patient underwent a first revision with caudal extension (2011). In June 2015 the hardware was completely removed for unknown reasons, and the next November the patient underwent a T7–T9 corpectomy with a mesh cage. In December 2015, the posterior instrumentation was extended caudally to L2. After this long list of repeated surgeries, the patient came to our attention complaining of coronal malalignment and poor sitting balance, together with back pain. The clinical examination showed left coronal malalignment, rod prominence in the lumbar area, and hypokyphosis in the thoracic area (**Fig. 16.1**).

In October 2016 the patient underwent surgical revision with posterior hardware removal, new fixation of T6–T11, and Smith-Petersen

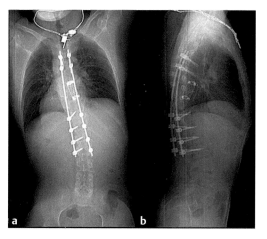

Fig. 16.1 Anteroposterior (AP) **(a)** and lateral (LL) **(b)** radiographs with the patient in the sitting position, showing left coronal malalignment and caudal instrumentation failure.

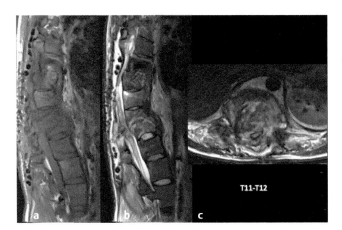

Fig. 16.2 Sagittal magnetic resonance imaging T1- **(a)** and T2-weighted **(b)** and T2 axial **(c)** scans, showing T11-T12 pyogenic diskitis.

osteotomies at T12-L1 and L1-L2. The goals of the surgery were to leave the thoracolumbar junction free to compensate and to eliminate the coronal malalignment.

On postoperative day 10, G.C. was readmitted from the rehabilitation center with a diagnosis of deep wound infection and sepsis. Blood cultures were positive for methicillin-resistant *S. aureus* (MRSA). Surgical washout and debridement were immediately performed, and the intraoperative samples confirmed the pathogen. Contact isolation and targeted antibiotic therapy were started, based on international guidelines. Sepsis progression, with high and increasing CRP levels and worsening clinical signs and symptoms (hypotension, lymphopenia, poor general condition) led to the decision to perform a second surgical washout and global hardware removal. After that, the clinical and laboratory parameters of infection did not improve. Intraoperative samples and MRI findings led to the diagnosis of T11-T12 infection sustained by MRSA (**Fig. 16.2**). Thus, a third surgery was performed, with T11-T12 corpectomy, deep washout and debridement, implant of a mesh cage, and posterior fixation extended to L2 (**Fig. 16.3**). After that, the patient showed improvement. Clinical and laboratory parameters slowly but progressively normalized. The patient's sitting balance was finally improved, he had a complete recovery in 1 month. The overall duration of antibiotic suppressive therapy was 8 weeks intravenous.

Although this case was successfully resolved, it is difficult to estimate the emotional, financial, and technical costs of such a life-threatening condition. The medical and surgical efforts were finally rewarded, but it seems more likely that patient-related factors played a major role. The following section discusses the impact of these factors on infection risk and successful treatment.

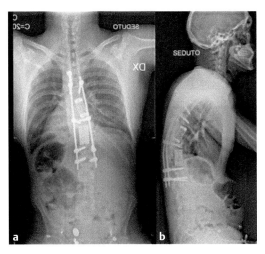

Fig. 16.3 Final postoperative sitting AP **(a)** and LL **(b)** radiographs, showing a mesh cage and posterior fixation to L2.

Risk Factors for Peri-Implant Postoperative Infections

After a careful review of the literature and a multivariate analysis, we determined that there are four independent risk factors for postoperative infection in adult instrumented spine surgery[28–30]:

1. Blood loss greater than 1 L, which entails a blood transfusion and subsequent immunosuppression, with an increased infection risk. Blood loss often correlates with a longer operative time.
2. Posterior approach, which is chosen for anatomic reasons. It entails better lymphatic and vascular drainage of the anterior spine.
3. Diabetes, which is a known risk factor, secondary to microangiopathy. Strict perioperative glycemic control ensures a better outcome in these patients.
4. Previous surgical infection, because even in the absence of clinical evidence of infection, some encapsulated bacteria can be reactivated due to surgical stress.

With a univariate analysis, several other important risk factors are identified:

- Obesity
- Inflammatory arthritis undergoing immunomodulating therapy
- Chronic steroid administration
- Cigarette smoking
- Parkinson's disease
- Malnutrition

It is difficult to summarize the evidence, as some results are biased by patient selection and by study design (retrospective in most cases). The above list is based on the findings of Pull ter Gunne and colleagues,[28,29] who published some of the best systematic reviews on the topic. One finding pertains to surveillance: greater attention should be paid to patients who present one or more of these risk factors.

We believe that malnutrition is an especially important factor. It is now evident that low serum albumin levels are strongly predictive of postoperative infection after spinal instrumented surgery.[31–33] Several parameters associated with malnutrition have been investigated. Serum albumin is usually dosed in a preoperative laboratory assessment of the patient. Low levels of this protein can be related to a systemic inflammatory state, a common situation in obese patients. Hypoalbuminemia is frequently found in both obese and underweight patients. This finding prompted research into the factors that can identify malnutrition with morphological and laboratory tests or with patient questionnaires. No consensus has been achieved, but research is continuing. In the meantime, greater attention should be paid to frail and malnourished patients in the postoperative period, and adequate protein support should be provided.

In our experience, patients with Parkinson's disease are at higher risk for peri-implant infections. A recent study found that Parkinson's disease is a predictor of major postoperative complications, including infections.[34]

Systemic and Local Antibiotics Administration

There is intense debate on the effectiveness of postoperative suppressive antibiotic treatment in peri-implant spinal infections. Even if there is some evidence that precludes its prolonged use, some systemic complications require intravenous administration of antibiotics. In most of the published studies, the postoperative care of patients with peri-implant infections is based on a targeted antibiotic therapy, with early intravenous administration for 4 to 8 weeks, and prolonged oral administration for a further 6 weeks to 3 months. Depending on the pathogen and the response, this suppressive therapy continued for more than 6 months in some studies. Keller and colleagues[35] found that suppressive antibiotic therapy in the first 3 months after debridement with implant retention fosters improved healing at 1-year follow-up.

Thus, there is no need for implant removal, significantly reducing the patient's morbidity and discomfort.

The empiric antibiotic protocol that we use in the early stage of the infection, just after the surgical debridement but before the microbiology results, is a combination of either vancomycin and meropenem or vancomycin and rifampin, depending on various patient factors and comorbidities, and on our clinical suspicion regarding the presence of specific pathogens. Close collaboration with infectious disease specialists is mandatory in determining the antibiotic protocol, because geographical and hospital-specific epidemiological criteria must be followed in fighting the drug resistance.

Local vancomycin administration during surgery is controversial. A literature review reported mixed results,[36] but a retrospective cohort comparative study (level of evidence: 3) recommends its use.[37] In our practice, after debridement, we apply bioactive glass to the infected bone surface, as it inhibits bacterial growth by osmotic and acid-base mechanisms.[38]

Antibiotic loaded cement scaffolds can be an interesting option in the treatment of severe spinal postsurgical osteomyelitis. The experience of bone-loaded cement comes from prosthetic infections, and it is well established in infections after hip and knee arthroplasty.[39,40] The main indication is in cases of two-stage revision surgery,[41] when the primary surgical revision is at high risk of re-infection or when anatomic conditions are not favorable for implant exchange. Antibiotic loaded spacers provide temporary support, reduce the dead space, maintain soft tissue tension and shape, provide gradual release of antibiotics, and have a positive impact on patients' symptoms.[42] Masuda and colleagues[43] analyzed the effect of antibiotic-loaded cement in postsurgical spinal infections refractory to standard care, and reported interesting results with complete healing and fusion in all cases, with surgical revision needed in fewer than 10% of cases. The main disadvantages and risks are related to the slow release of antibiotics, the risk of resistance selection of bacteria, and the risk of polymethylmethacrylate (PMMA) becoming a focus of secondary colonization if it is not removed.

Wound Management and Care

Wound management is critical in postoperative spinal infections, especially when multiple debridement procedures are performed. Soft tissues are usually harvested, resulting in a space in which fluids can collect. Fluid collection in this dead, hypovascular space is a likely medium for bacterial growth, thereby increasing the risk of bacterial regrowth. The use of vacuum-assisted closure (VAC) aims to reduce fluid collection and dead space, producing a continuous negative pressure and allowing fluid suction outside the wound, with a close system. Continuous drainage prevents bacterial growth and colony formation and provides a mechanical stimulus for soft tissue regeneration and healing.[44–46] Although evidence is lacking regarding the cost-effectiveness of the primary use of VAC in instrumented spine surgery, VAC is probably the best way to manage infected wounds after repeated debridement, enabling implant retention. Plastic surgery studies have provided evidence that, in cases of complex wounds, VAC closures result in shorter hospital stays and a faster wound healing.[47,48] The main risk factor for VAC failure is bacteria. The presence of multiresistant staphylococci frequently results in the failure of both conservative treatment and VAC dressing management of the wound.

In such difficult and refractory cases, further surgeries are often performed, with repeated stress on skin and subcutaneous tissue. In cases of skin and subcutaneous tissue necrosis and defect, a surgical flap could be the solution.[49–51] In cases of small superficial skin defects, a simple skin flap can be sufficient. Unfortunately, in cases of severe infections, the soft tissue defect can be extensive and severe. In these cases, muscle flaps are the best choice. They provide bone and soft tissue coverage with dead space filling, they provide vascularity with oxygen and white and red blood cells for the immune response against bacteria, and they deliver antibiotics.

A plastic surgeon should always be consulted when a large soft tissue defect is addressed. The choice of the flap is based on several technical and patient-related factors, and appropriate preoperative planning is required for a successful surgical repair. Muscular flaps are mandatory in cases of hardware exposure or exposure of the dural sac.

Wound management is critical in repeated debridement. Vacuum-assisted closure is a useful tool to prevent dead space and fluid collection, especially in cases of repeated debridement with hardware retention. In cases of hardware exposure or dural sac exposure, or in cases of large soft tissue defects, muscle flaps are the best solution.

▣ Chapter Summary

Infections in the postoperative instrumented spine are an unpredictable, severe complication, with significant morbidity and mortality. Early detection and aggressive treatment are the hallmarks of a successful outcome. Infection onset can be early or delayed, requiring specific bacteriology and pharmacological management. *Staphylococcus aureus* is most frequently isolated from cultures. The instrumentation can be retained successfully in most cases of early infection, but, in some delayed presentations, hardware removal is the only way to eradicate the infection. This is probably due to the presence of a structured biofilm.

It is possible to identify patients at high risk for postoperative infections, as patient-related factors are the most important predictors of the final outcome, regardless of the duration of antibiotic therapy and the success of the surgical debridement. Recent studies confirm that poor nutritional status is one of the strongest risk factors for postoperative infection in instrumented spine surgery.

Pearls

◆ Early identification of infection is the key for successful treatment while retaining the instrumentation.
◆ Early, aggressive treatment with surgical debridement is mandatory.
◆ In delayed infections, it is frequently necessary to remove the implant to achieve complete eradication.
◆ MRI is the imaging modality of choice in the evaluation of peri-implant infection.
◆ C-reactive protein is a reliable marker for the diagnosis and monitoring of infection during antibiotic therapy.

Pitfalls

◆ The type and duration of systemic antibiotic targeted therapy must be carefully evaluated in consultation with an infectious disease specialist.
◆ In the presence of delayed infection, it may be prudent to avoid removal of the implant in patients who had undergone surgery with severe instability, such as three-column osteotomies.
◆ Poor nutritional status is a strong risk factor for postoperative infection. For these patients, consider prescribing a nutritional preparation before surgery, especially in nonemergency cases.

References
Five Must-Read References

1. McClelland S III, Takemoto RC, Lonner BS, et al. Analysis of postoperative thoracolumbar spine infections in a prospective randomized controlled trial using the centers for disease control surgical site infection criteria. Int J Spine Surg 2016; 10:14

2. Patel H, Khoury H, Girgenti D, Welner S, Yu H. Burden of surgical site infections associated with select spine operations and involvement of Staphylococcus aureus. Surg Infect (Larchmt) 2016

3. Nota SP, Braun Y, Ring D, Schwab JH. Incidence of surgical site infection after spine surgery: what is the impact of the definition of infection? Clin Orthop Relat Res 2015;473:1612–1619

4. Smith JS, Shaffrey CI, Sansur CA, et al; Scoliosis Research Society Morbidity and Mortality Committee. Rates of infection after spine surgery based on 108,419 procedures: a report from the Scoliosis Research Society Morbidity and Mortality Committee. Spine 2011;36:556–563

5. Shaffer WO, Baisden JL, Fernand R, Matz PG; North American Spine Society. An evidence-based clinical guideline for antibiotic prophylaxis in spine surgery. Spine J 2013;13:1387–1392

6. Cowperthwaite L, Holm RL. Guideline implementation: preoperative patient skin antisepsis. AORN J 2015;101:71–77, quiz 78–80

7. Anderson DJ, Podgorny K, Berríos-Torres SI, et al. Strategies to prevent surgical site infections in acute care hospitals: 2014 update. Infect Control Hosp Epidemiol 2014;35:605–627

8. Cunningham ME, Girardi F, Papadopoulos EC, Cammisa FP. Spinal infections in patients with compromised immune systems. Clin Orthop Relat Res 2006;444:73–82

9. Abdul-Jabbar A, Takemoto S, Weber MH, et al. Surgical site infection in spinal surgery: description of surgical and patient-based risk factors for postoperative infection using administrative claims data. Spine 2012;37:1340–1345

10. Hahn F, Zbinden R, Min K. Late implant infections caused by Propionibacterium acnes in scoliosis surgery. Eur Spine J 2005;14:783–788

11. Stinchfield FE, Bigliani LU, Neu HC, Goss TP, Foster CR. Late hematogenous infection of total joint replacement. J Bone Joint Surg Am 1980;62:1345–1350

12. Watters W III, Rethman MP, Hanson NB, et al; American Academy of Orthopaedic Surgeons; American Dental Association. Prevention of orthopaedic implant infection in patients undergoing dental procedures. J Am Acad Orthop Surg 2013;21:180–189

13. Lewkonia P, DiPaola C, Street J. Incidence and risk of delayed surgical site infection following instrumented lumbar spine fusion. J Clin Neurosci 2016;23:76–80

14. Kasliwal MK, Tan LA, Traynelis VC. Infection with spinal instrumentation: review of pathogenesis, diagnosis, prevention, and management. Surg Neurol Int 2013;4(Suppl 5):S392–S403

15. Lall RR, Wong AP, Lall RR, Lawton CD, Smith ZA, Dahdaleh NS. Evidence-based management of deep wound infection after spinal instrumentation. J Clin Neurosci 2015;22:238–242

16. Picada R, Winter RB, Lonstein JE, et al. Postoperative deep wound infection in adults after posterior lumbosacral spine fusion with instrumentation: incidence and management. J Spinal Disord 2000;13:42–45

17. Lian XF, Xu JG, Zeng BF, et al. Continuous irrigation and drainage for early postoperative deep wound infection after posterior instrumented spinal fusion. J Spinal Disord Tech 2014;27:E315–E317

18. Wille H, Dauchy FA, Desclaux A, et al. Efficacy of debridement, antibiotic therapy and implant retention within three months during postoperative instrumented spine infections. Infect Dis (Lond) 2017;49:261–267

19. Maruo K, Berven SH. Outcome and treatment of postoperative spine surgical site infections: predictors of treatment success and failure. J Orthop Sci 2014;19:398–404

20. Kowalski TJ, Berbari EF, Huddleston PM, Steckelberg JM, Mandrekar JN, Osmon DR. The management and outcome of spinal implant infections: contemporary retrospective cohort study. Clin Infect Dis 2007;44:913–920

21. Ahmed R, Greenlee JD, Traynelis VC. Preservation of spinal instrumentation after development of postoperative bacterial infections in patients undergoing spinal arthrodesis. J Spinal Disord Tech 2012;25:299–302

22. Kanayama M, Hashimoto T, Shigenobu K, Oha F, Iwata A, Tanaka M. MRI-based decision making of implant removal in deep wound infection after instrumented lumbar fusion. Clin Spine Surg 2017;30:E99–E103

23. Hedequist D, Haugen A, Hresko T, Emans J. Failure of attempted implant retention in spinal deformity delayed surgical site infections. Spine 2009;34:60–64

24. Ho C, Skaggs DL, Weiss JM, Tolo VT. Management of infection after instrumented posterior spine fusion in pediatric scoliosis. Spine 2007;32:2739–2744

25. Richards BR, Emara KM. Delayed infections after posterior TSRH spinal instrumentation for idiopathic scoliosis: revisited. Spine 2001;26:1990–1996

26. Tominaga H, Setoguchi T, Ishidou Y, Nagano S, Yamamoto T, Komiya S. Risk factors for surgical site infection and urinary tract infection after spine surgery. Eur Spine J 2016;25:3908–3915

27. DiPaola CP, Saravanja DD, Boriani L, et al. Postoperative infection treatment score for the spine (PITSS): construction and validation of a predictive model to define need for single versus multiple irrigation and debridement for spinal surgical site infection. Spine J 2012;12:218–230

28. Pull ter Gunne AF, Cohen DB. Incidence, prevalence, and analysis of risk factors for surgical site infection following adult spinal surgery. Spine 2009;34:1422–1428

29. Pull ter Gunne AF, Hosman AJ, Cohen DB, et al. A methodological systematic review on surgical site infections following spinal surgery: part 1: risk factors. Spine 2012;37:2017–2033

30. Xing D, Ma JX, Ma XL, Song DH, Wang J, Chen Y, et al. A methodological, systematic review of evidence-based independent risk factors for surgical site infections after spinal surgery. Eur Spine J 2013;22:605–615

31. Bohl DD, Shen MR, Mayo BC, et al. Malnutrition predicts infectious and wound complications following posterior lumbar spinal fusion. Spine 2016;41:1693–1699

32. Iwata E, Shigematsu H, Okuda A, et al. Lymphopenia at 4 days postoperatively is the most significant labo-

ratory marker for early detection of surgical site infection following posterior lumbar instrumentation surgery. Asian Spine J 2016;10:1042–1046

33. Kudo D, Miyakoshi N, Hongo M, Kasukawa Y, Ishikawa Y, Mizutani T, et al. Relationship between preoperative serum rapid turnover proteins and early-stage surgical wound infection after spine surgery. Eur Spine J 2017;26:3156–3161

34. Oichi T, Chikuda H, Ohya J, et al. Mortality and morbidity after spinal surgery in patients with Parkinson disease: a retrospective matched-pair cohort study. Spine J 2016

35. Keller SC, Cosgrove SE, Higgins Y, Piggott DA, Osgood G, Auwaerter PG. Role of suppressive oral antibiotics in orthopedic hardware infections for those not undergoing two-stage replacement surgery. Open Forum Infect Dis 2016;3:ofw176

36. Khan NR, Thompson CJ, DeCuypere M, et al. A meta-analysis of spinal surgical site infection and vancomycin powder. J Neurosurg Spine 2014;21:974–983

37. Hey HW, Thiam DW, Koh ZS, et al. Is intraoperative local vancomycin powder the answer to surgical site infections in spine surgery? Spine 2017;42:267–274

38. Drago L, Vassena C, Fenu S, et al. In vitro antibiofilm activity of bioactive glass S53P4. Future Microbiol 2014;9:593–601

39. Helbig L, Bechberger M, Aldeeri R, et al. Initial peri- and postoperative antibiotic treatment of infected nonunions: results from 212 consecutive patients after mean follow-up of 34 months. Ther Clin Risk Manag 2018;14:59–67

40. Grubhofer F, Imam MA, Wieser K, Achermann Y, Meyer DC, Gerber C. Staged revision with antibiotic spacers for shoulder prosthetic joint infections yields high infection control. Clin Orthop Relat Res 2018; 476:146–152

41. Anagnostakos K, Fink B. Antibiotic-loaded cement spacers - lessons learned from the past 20 years. Expert Rev Med Devices 2018;15:231–245

42. Fleck EE, Spangehl MJ, Rapuri VR, Beauchamp CP. An articulating antibiotic spacer controls infection and improves pain and function in a degenerative

septic hip. Clin Orthop Relat Res 2011;469:3055–3064

43. Masuda S, Fujibayashi S, Otsuki B, Kimura H, Matsuda S. Efficacy of target drug delivery and dead space reduction using antibiotic-loaded bone cement for the treatment of complex spinal infection. Clin Spine Surg 2017;30:E1246–E1250

44. Mehbod AA, Ogilvie JW, Pinto MR, et al. Postoperative deep wound infections in adults after spinal fusion: management with vacuum-assisted wound closure. J Spinal Disord Tech 2005;18:14–17

45. Watt JP, Dunn RN. The use of vacuum dressings for dead space management in deep surgical site infections allows implant and bone graft retention. Global Spine J 2017;7:756–761

46. Ploumis A, Mehbod AA, Dressel TD, Dykes DC, Transfeldt EE, Lonstein JE. Therapy of spinal wound infections using vacuum-assisted wound closure: risk factors leading to resistance to treatment. J Spinal Disord Tech 2008;21:320–323

47. de Laat EH, van den Boogaard MH, Spauwen PH, van Kuppevelt DH, van Goor H, Schoonhoven L. Faster wound healing with topical negative pressure therapy in difficult-to-heal wounds: a prospective randomized controlled trial. Ann Plast Surg 2011;67: 626–631

48. Ozden R, Duman IG, Uruc V, Dogramaci Y, Kalaci A, Komurcu E. The comparison of vacuum assisted closure and conventional cotton gauze dressing in the treatment of defective lower extremity injuries. Acta Med Mediter 2014;30:1337–1342

49. Rubayi S, Chandrasekhar BS. Trunk, abdomen, and pressure sore reconstruction. Plast Reconstr Surg 2011;128:201e–215e

50. Brown NL, Rose MB, Blueschke G, et al. Bioburden after Staphylococcus aureus inoculation in type 1 diabetic rats undergoing internal fixation. Plast Reconstr Surg 2014;134:412e–419e

51. Dumanian GA. Discussion: immediate soft-tissue reconstruction for complex defects of the spine following surgery for spinal neoplasms. Plast Reconstr Surg 2010;125:1467–1468

17

Spinal Infections in Geriatric Patients

Yoshiharu Kawaguchi

Introduction

The spine is a common site of musculoskeletal infections. Spinal infection encompasses pyogenic spondylodiskitis, vertebral osteomyelitis, epidural abscess, and iliopsoas abscess. The disease causes not only local symptoms, such as back pain, leg pain, and neurologic deficit, but also deterioration of the patient's general condition, which is evident in such symptoms as general malaise, fever, and vital organ failure due to sepsis. Spinal infection is a life-threatening disease. Several studies[1–7] reviewed spinal infection and discussed the management of spinal infection, as it is an important disease entity worldwide. This chapter focuses on the clinical characteristics, diagnosis, and treatment of spinal infection in geriatric patients.

Epidemiology

The estimated incidence of spinal infection is reported to range from 1 in 40,000 to 1 in 250,000 population per year.[8] The Japanese Survey for Vertebral Osteomyelitis, using the Japanese Diagnosis Procedure Combination Database, reported that the estimated incidence of vertebral osteomyelitis has gradually increased in recent years.[8] This survey reported an incidence of 5.3 in 100,000 population per

year in 2007, increasing to 6.3 in 2008, 7.1 in 2009, and 7.4 in 2010. The same increasing tendency was evident from the data from 1995 to 2008 in Denmark.[9] It has also been evident in Japanese studies that the incidence markedly increases with age among people 60 to 80 years of age.[8,9] The incidence per 100,000 population per year in patients younger than 59 was 1.7, whereas in those aged 60 to 69 years it was 10.9, in those aged 70 to 79 years it was 21.6, and in those 80 or older it was 25.1.[8] The incidence was 9.8 in 100,000 per year in New Zealand for those aged > 65 years,[10] and it was the highest in Denmark in those aged > 70 years.[11] Geriatric patients commonly have comorbidity related to their general condition. In the survey of Carragee,[6] the patients with pyogenic vertebral osteomyelitis were older and more likely to have a comorbid condition than was previously reported.

As for surgical site infection (SSI) in spine surgery, the Japanese Society for Spine Surgery–Related Research (JSSR) reported that the incidence of deep wound infection was 1.4% in 8,033 patients who had spine surgery.[12] Another multicenter study in Japan reported that the incidence of complications was significantly higher in patients older than 65 years, including SSI.[13] Several studies have shown that geriatric patients are more prone to SSI in spine surgery.[14,15] This might be caused by immune deficiency in geriatric patients.

Pathology

Primarily, bacteremia causes hematogenous infection of the spine. There are two major routes for hematogenous dissemination of bacteria: venous and arterial. Wiley and Trueta[16] suggested that bacteria can become lodged in the arteriolar network at the vertebral end plate. Batson has demonstrated retrograde flow of veins from the pelvic venous plexus to the perivertebral plexus which has been confirmed in other studies as well.[17] The infection in the pelvis or urinary tract may be spread via Batson plexus routes. The main focus of spinal infection is the intervertebral disk (IVD) in adults. The IVD is avascular, and bacteria invades the end-arterial arcades in the metaphyseal region adjacent to the IVD. The infection then spreads by direct extension, with rupture of the infective lesion through the end plate into the IVD. It may extend from the vertebral body to the subligamentous paravertebral area, the epidural space and contiguous vertebral bodies.[18] The other route is direct invasion from the needle at diskography. Diskitis after diskography is due to bacterial penetration into the IVD by a contaminated needle. The incidence of diskitis from diskography was reported to be 1 to 4%.[19] One case report found a pyogenic spondylodiskitis due to *Pseudomonas aeruginosa* after computed tomography (CT)-guided facet joint steroid injection in a 78-year-old man.[20]

Hematogenous vertebral osteomyelitis is generally a single bacterial infection,[21] although the pathogenic bacteria may not always be detected. This is especially common when antibiotics are used before examinations for the detection of bacteria. Many studies demonstrated that *Staphylococcus aureus* is the most commonly isolated bacteria.[1,22,23] Although *S. aureus* accounts for more than 50% of isolates, the diversity of causative bacteria is wide.[1] In a study on vertebral osteomyelitis in geriatric patients, a shift in the frequency distribution of pathogens to gram-negative bacteria, such as *Escherichia coli*, has been observed. Belzunegui et al[24] reported that *E. coli* was isolated in seven of 34 elderly patients and in none of 38 young patients. This might be characteristic of

elderly men who have a history of urinary tract infection. However, Sobottke et al[23] stated that the most frequent pathogen identified in 50% of cases was *S. aureus*. They did not see a shift to gram-negative pathogens in their study, which was focused on spondylodiskitis in elderly patients.

Clinical Features

The diagnosis of pyogenic spinal infection is based on clinical symptoms, radiological findings, and microbiological analyses. Local pain, usually back pain, is the most common symptom, with a prevalence of more than 90% of the patients with pyogenic spinal infection. This might be due to destruction of the vertebral structure or pressure rendered by the abscess. However, as this is not a specific clinical symptom, a delay in diagnosis is not uncommon. Especially in geriatric patients, it might be erroneously assumed that the pain is caused by degenerative spinal change. In addition, the presence of comorbidities such as diabetes can result in less severe constitutional symptoms. Thus, it takes from 2 to 12 weeks and occasionally more than 3 months before the diagnosis is made.[23] Fever is thought to be associated with infection, but it is typically not present and it accounts for less than 20% of infections. This is usually true even in geriatric patients. Other symptoms such as anorexia, general malaise, and weight loss are also not specific to spinal infection. Neurologic deficit might be caused when an epidural abscess compresses the spinal cord, cauda equina, or spinal nerves. However, the incidence of motor palsy by spinal infection is less common. Butler et al[25] reported that 27% of patients with infective spondylitis had neurologic involvement requiring surgical intervention. Most of these patients had an incomplete neurologic deficit with mild extremity motor weakness; this might be one reason for the delay in the diagnosis, as physicians might assume that the weakness is caused by general malaise or disuse in geriatric patients with spinal infection, even though spinal infection associated with epidural abscess causes a neurologic deficit. However, in a retrospective study, Eismont et al[26] reported that old age as well as the associated diseases of diabetes mellitus and rheumatoid arthritis and a more cephalad level of infection were the predisposing factors to paralysis.

Geriatric patients tend to have comorbidities. In some cases, geriatric patients develop spondylodiskitis from a primary focus infection elsewhere, such as urinary tract infection or pneumonia. Symptoms related to spondylodiskitis should be sought. Further, preexisting neurologic conditions such as sensorimotor neuropathy, motor neuron disease, and Parkinson's disease can mask typical neurologic symptoms, and, contrarily, the neurologic symptoms of neural compression can be mistaken for diabetic neuropathy. Therefore, special attention should be paid to patients with these conditions.

Diagnosis

Laboratory Data

Laboratory markers, such as white blood cell (WBC) count, C-reactive protein (CRP), and erythrocyte sedimentation rate (ESR), are well-known inflammatory biomarkers for infection, although they are not specific for spinal infection.[1,3] An elevation in these markers should not be taken as pathognomonic for an infection, but these markers serve as good screening and surveillance examinations in the diagnosis and treatment of spinal infection. Among the three biomarkers, Yee et al[27] assessed the relationship between both presentation and peak value and age in patients with pyogenic spondylosis who were intravenous drug users. In their results, the WBC count on presentation for patients 65 years of age or older was significantly higher than in those younger than 65 years of age; in contrast, there was no significant difference in ESR and CRP. Further, there was no significant difference in the peak values of these markers between the patients > 65 years old and the younger patients.

Recently, procalcitonin (PCT) has been used to distinguish bacterial infection from nonbacterial infection. Jeong et al[28] examined the clinical value of PCT in patients with spinal infection and found that the sensitivity of PCT was lower than that of CRP. Based on these results, they concluded that patients with spinal infection who showed an elevated serum PCT level should be examined for combined infection, and that antibiotics targeted to spinal infection and to the other combined infection should be prescribed. Yoon et al[29] reported that a combination of clinical data and biomarkers had better predictive value for differential diagnosis compared with biomarkers alone in their multicenter study for infectious spondylodiskitis.

It is important to perform urine and blood cultures to identify the organism when infection is highly probable, although the rate of identification of the organism is not very high. Prophylactic use of antibiotics usually masks the presence of the organism. It is also essential to check for anemia, albumin (malnutrition), and liver function status in the management of spinal infection in geriatric patients.

Imaging Studies

Imaging studies are very important for the diagnosis of spinal infection. They include plain radiographs, CT, magnetic resonance imaging (MRI), ^{18}F-fluorodeoxyglucose–positron emission tomography (FDG-PET), scintigraphy, and single photon emission computed tomography (SPECT). There are no typical image findings in geriatric patients with spinal infection. The findings are relatively dependent on the stage of the disease.

Plain radiographs should be the first imaging study in all patients suspected of having spinal infection. They demonstrate various findings based on the stage of spinal infection. Plain radiographs are also suitable for follow-up study. At the early stage, 2 to 8 weeks after the onset of the infection, end-plate irregularity and disk space narrowing are found. After 8 to 12 weeks, bone destruction might be observed, which results in changes in spinal alignment. Spinal infection sometimes causes local kyphotic deformity, which can rapidly progress in geriatric patients who have severe osteoporosis. The presence of preexisting spinal degeneration, diffuse idiopathic skeletal hyperostosis (DISH), osteoporosis, spondylolisthesis, and spinal stenosis should also be determined in radiographs. These conditions can help determine the type of management and the approach for surgical treatment. Plain radiographs can also demonstrate soft tissue swelling, suggesting paraspinal abscess.

Computed tomography is used for the examination of bone destruction as well as soft tissue swelling. A moth-eaten appearance at both end plates on the affected IVD is seen in spondylodiskitis (**Fig. 17.1a–c**). CT is commonly used for image-guided biopsy.

Magnetic resonance imaging (MRI) is the gold standard for diagnosing spinal infection. It is more useful for the detection of spinal infection at an early stage, as compared with plain radiographs and CT. The sensitivity, specificity, and accuracy of MRI are reported to be 96%, 92%, and 94%, respectively, which are very high.[30] However, care must be taken in the interpretation of the MRI findings, because the presence of exuberant edema in adjacent zones may seem to indicate that the spinal infection covers a larger area than it does. The typical MRI pattern for the early stage of spinal infection is low intensity on T1-weighted imaging (T1 low) and high intensity on T2-weighted imaging (T2 high) at the IVD and the end plates (**Fig. 17.1d,e**). This finding suggests a fluid signal caused by bone edema. A mirror image, which shows upper and lower end-plate damage at the affected IVD level, can be seen on T1 and T2 MRI in patients with spinal infection. T2 high is sometimes clearly observed at the IVD. This suggests degradation of the IVD by the enzyme from bacteria. On the other hand, a metastatic lesion is often seen in the bone

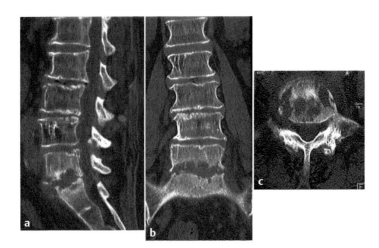

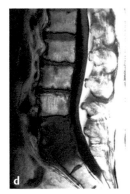
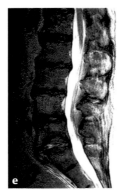

Fig. 17.1 An 82-year-old woman presented with L5-S1 spondylodiskitis. Computed tomography (CT) images: **(a)** sagittal view, **(b)** frontal view, and **(c)** axial view at the L5-S1 level. The moth-eaten appearance is clearly seen at the L5-S1 level, suggesting infection at this level. Magnetic resonance imaging (MRI), sagittal **(d)** T1-weighted imaging and **(e)** T2-weighted imaging. T1 low and T2 high was clearly observed at L5-S1, suggesting L5-S1 spondylodiskitis.

structure, such as the vertebral body and pedicle. The metastatic lesion occurs through blood flow; thus, the metastatic lesion preserves the structure of the IVD, as the IVD is an avascular tissue. This is a characteristic finding in the differential diagnosis between infectious and metastatic lesions in the spine.

Magnetic resonance imaging is the best noninvasive imaging tool to assess the spread of infection to the epidural space. An epidural abscess causes a neurologic deficit associated with intolerable local pain. The detection of the epidural abscess is very important for predicting the symptoms and also to determine the treatment. T1-gadolinium–enhanced MRI is sometimes useful for the detection of an epidural abscess.

Degenerative end-plate changes seen in MRI are called as Modic signs, which can sometimes be confused with spinal infections (**Fig. 17.2**). Modic signs are of three types[31]: type 1 shows T1 low and T2 high, corresponding to vertebral body edema and hypervascularity; type 2 shows T1 high and T2 high, reflecting fatty replacements of red bone marrow; type 3 shows T1 low and T2 low, suggestive of subchondral bone sclerosis. Modic type 2 is most frequently seen, followed by Modic type 1 and then Modic type 3. Interestingly, some studies suggest that Modic type 1 is associated with infection. Albert et al[32] reported that treatment with anti-biotics (amoxicillin-clavulanate) is effective in Modic type 1 patients with lower back pain (LBP). Ohtori et al[33] followed 71 patients with Modic type 1 for 2 years and found that three patients had a spinal infection that was found later, which might imply that some Modic type 1 patients have a hypovirulent infection, especially at the end plate. Other studies have demonstrated that FDG-PET or diffusion MRI might be useful for the detection of infection in patients with Modic type 1.[34,35] More evidence should be collected to confirm these findings. **Table 17.1** lists the differential diagnosis of spondylodiskitis, spinal metastasis, and osteoporotic vertebral fracture using MRI findings.

[18]F-fluorodeoxyglucose–positron emission tomography is a three-dimensional imaging tool. ^{18}F-fluorodeoxyglucose has increased uptake in tissue that is active for metabolism, such as malignant tumor and infection. The usefulness of FDG-PET has been shown in musculoskeletal infection, including spinal infection. A meta-analysis regarding FDG-PET as a diagnostic tool of spinal infection reported that the sensitivity was 97% and specificity was 88%; the positive predictive value was 0.96 and negative predictive value was 0.85.[36]

Scintigraphy has been frequently used as a diagnostic tool for spinal infection as well as bone metastasis. Bone scan employing technetium 99m as the radioisotope-labeled tracer is useful for the detection of infection at the early stage. Gallium 67 is also used for the analysis of infection. These are two-dimensional imaging studies. SPECT is a three-dimensional imaging study. In the comparison between bone scan and SPECT, SPECT had higher sensitivity and specificity. It has been reported that SPECT detected an additional 30% of solitary vertebral lesions in patients with LBP.[37]

Biopsy

It is very important to determine the causative organism of the infection. If the patient has sepsis with a high-grade fever, a blood culture should be attempted. If the blood culture is negative, a local biopsy should be performed, such as a fluoroscope- or CT-guided percutaneous biopsy. The accuracy of a percutaneous ver-

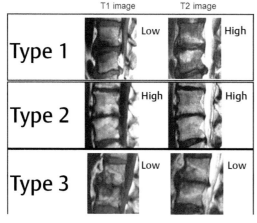

Fig. 17.2 Modic signs, types 1, 2, and 3. See the text (Diagnosis: Image Section) for a description of the three types.

Table 17.1 Differential Diagnosis Including Spondylodiskitis, Spinal Metastasis, and Osteoporotic Vertebral Fracture Using Magnetic Resonance Imaging (MRI) Findings

Abnormal Finding in MRI	Spondylodiskitis	Spinal Metastasis	Osteoporotic Vertebral Fracture
End-plate irregularity	+	–	–
Disk space narrowing	+	–	–
T2 high intensity in the disk	+	–	–
Mirror image in adjacent vertebral bodies	+	–	–
Paravertebral abscess	+	–	–
Spot lesion in vertebral body	–	+	–
Focal destruction of vertebral body	–	+	–
Diffuse destruction of vertebral body	±	+	+
Collapse of vertebral body	±	+	+
General osteoporosis	±	±	+
Wedged vertebrae	±	±	+

tebral biopsy in patients with spinal infection is 70%.[3] Negative results may be caused by an insufficient sample or the administration of antibiotics before the biopsy. Biopsy is an invasive diagnostic method, and therefore care must be taken in geriatric patients, especially with those on anticoagulant medications.

▨ Treatment

The goal of treatment is to cure the infection, prevent relapse, control pain, and restore function. Nonoperative treatment, using antibiotics and immobilization of the area with the infective lesion, is tried first, as most patients with spinal infection can be treated conservatively.

Conservative Treatment

When the bacteria is determined, the appropriate antibiotic, with a high bioavailability in the bone, is prescribed. Nickerson and Sinha[1] summarized the recommendations for specific intravenous antibiotics for the identified common causes of pyogenic vertebral osteomyelitis from pooled reviews. However, it is difficult to select an appropriate antibiotic when the bacteria is not determined. In that case, broad-spectrum antibiotics that cover *S. au-*

reus should be used as empirical treatment, as *S. aureus* is the most common cause of spinal infection.[22,23] In the case of an immunocompromised host, one might suggest the use of broad-spectrum antibiotics along with and a non–methicillin-resistant *S. aureus* (MRSA) drug, as antibiotic-resistant organisms, such as MRSA, are commonly isolated. Vancomycin is the first choice for MRSA infection. New agents, such as linezolid and daptomycin, have been recently used.

In geriatric patients, care must be taken to monitor their renal and liver function before, during, and after antibiotic treatment. There is no consensus regarding the duration of antibiotic treatment for spinal infection. A wide variation exists in the clinical use of antibiotics intravenously and orally. Cheung and Luk[3] reported that some authors recommend 6 to 8 weeks of intravenous antibiotic therapy and others recommend only 4 weeks. An open-label, noninferiority, randomized controlled trial published in Lancet in 2014 demonstrated that 6 weeks of antibiotic treatment is not inferior to 12 weeks of antibiotic treatment with respect to the numbers of patients with pyogenic vertebral osteomyelitis who are cured at 1 year.[38] Based on those results, the authors stated that the standard antibiotic treatment duration for patients with this disease could be reduced to 6 weeks.

Laboratory data and imaging studies are important for monitoring. CRP is more useful than ESR, because the elevation of ESR tends to be prolonged and ESR is affected by many factors that are not directly related to infection. Plain radiographs and MRI are recommended for the follow-up imaging study. CT is radiologically invasive. When spontaneous spinal fusion is achieved, the local pathology is considered to be healed.

Bed rest is recommended at the early phase of spinal infection, especially when the patient complains of severe local pain. However, bed rest itself results in disuse atrophy, especially for geriatric patients. Thus, immobilization of the spine using a corset is a standard clinical practice. We recommend a hard corset for more than 3 months for the treatment of lumbar spinal infection. However, there is no consensus regarding the duration of corset application.

Surgical Treatment

Although most spinal infection cases can be managed nonoperatively, 10 to 20% of patients require a surgical approach. The indications for surgery in vertebral osteomyelitis are (1) failure to respond to antimicrobial therapy/source control, (2) neurologic impairment or deterioration, (3) spinal instability or deformity that may result in intractable pain, (4) epidural abscesses and paraspinal abscesses (certainly ≥ 2.5 cm), and (5) significant vertebral destruction or impending fractures.[1] In particular, in patients with neurologic deficit due to epidural abscess, surgical treatment is absolutely indicated, because permanent neural deficit might occur in such cases.

Debridement of infected tissue, stabilization of the infected lesion and spinal reconstruction are mandatory for surgical management. Debridement is effective for reducing the bacteria in the lesion and also effective for creating the access route for antibiotics to reach the lesion. Percutaneous drainage or debridement has been introduced for spinal infection. This procedure might be considered in high-risk geriatric patients, as it is a minimally invasive method. Stabilization is needed to decrease the inflammation due to infection. Reconstruction prevents progressive deformity of the spinal alignment. Although recent reports support the use of internal fixation, the use of instrumentation for spinal infection is still controversial.[3] Internal fixation with instrumentation maintains spinal stability and alignment, prevents postoperative kyphotic deformity, and promotes bone fusion. The anterior approach, with meticulous debridement followed by anterior interbody fusion, is traditionally used in many cases, because the main focus of the spinal infection is within the anterior column of the spine. A surgical plan should be considered based on the condition of the osteoporosis, a preexisting degenerative olisthesis or spinal stenosis adjacent to the level of infection, and the presence of diffuse idiopathic spinal hyperostosis. The preferred surgical method at my center is anterior debridement plus interbody fusion with an autograft from the iliac crest, followed by posterior fixation with instrumentation. Titanium mesh cages are increasingly being used in infected lesions, as the cage resists bacterial adherence better than other materials. Several studies have reported that the use of metallic implants after radical debridement of the infected spine does not lead to the persistence or recurrence of the infection.[39,40] Spinal infection is judged to be healed when laboratory data become normalized and bone fusion is demonstrated by radiological examinations. Special attention should be paid to cases of fixation failure.

Surgical intervention might be questionable in geriatric patients who are in poor general condition. Similarly, surgeons might be reluctant to perform surgery in geriatric patients due to the high complication rate. However, Sobottke et al[23] have shown that advanced age is not associated with increased morbidity or mortality, and that operative results and complication rates are comparable in older and younger patients. Thus, these authors concluded that advanced age should not be a crucial factor in the decision making of surgical intervention in spinal infection. In contrast, another study reported that mortality in patients with spinal infection is significantly associated with comorbidity and advanced age.[8] The mortality rate in pyogenic vertebral osteomyelitis widely ranges from 4 to 29%.[1] Because the incidence of spinal infection increases with age and older patients tend to have comorbidities, special attention must be paid to the surgical management of geriatric patients with spinal infection.

Chapter Summary

This review clarifies the characteristics of spinal infection in geriatric patients. The following findings are important for the diagnosis and treatment of geriatric patients with spinal infection: (1) the diagnosis might be delayed because the symptoms of spinal infection are not specific and the physician tends to misinterpret the symptoms that are caused by degenerative spinal change; (2) old age is a predisposing factor for spinal infections because of immuno deficiency; (3) S. aureus is the most common bacteria that is identified in geriatric patients with spinal infection; (4) MRI is the gold standard for imaging diagnosis, although there is no specific finding in geriatric patients; (5) conservative treatment is primarily performed, and broad-spectrum antibiotics that cover S. aureus should be considered; (6) there is a paucity of data regarding the surgical complication rate in geriatric patients, but advanced age alone should not be a contraindication to surgical intervention. A recent study has reported that tubercular spondylodiskitis in elderly patients differed from that in younger patients because of the greater presence of comorbidities, the later presentation,

the greater neurologic deficit, the greater mortality, and increased complications.[41] Nevertheless, the authors emphasized that in those who survived, clinicoradiological outcomes of both conservative and surgical treatments were good.

Recent findings suggest that the incidence of spinal infection is increasing, especially in old patients. Prompt diagnosis and suitable treatment are important for spinal infection, especially in geriatric patients.

Pearls

- Diagnosis might be delayed because the symptoms of spinal infection are not specific, and physicians often misinterpret the symptoms that are caused by degenerative spinal change.
- *Staphylococcus aureus* is the most common bacteria identified in geriatric patients with spinal infection.
- Conservative treatment is primarily performed using broad-spectrum antibiotics, but surgical intervention should be considered in patients who have operative indications.

Pitfalls

- Consider spinal infection in geriatric patients who suffer from prolonged low back pain.
- Perform a biopsy to determine the organism that causes the spinal infection.
- Check the stage and the clinical course of the spinal infection using imaging studies.
- Proceed with the appropriate treatment for spinal infection, with conservative therapy using antibiotics alone in early cases and surgical therapy in late presentations with complications.

References

Five Must-Read References

1. Nickerson EK, Sinha R. Vertebral osteomyelitis in adults: an update. Br Med Bull 2016;117:121–138
2. Hopkinson N, Patel K. Clinical features of septic discitis in the UK: a retrospective case ascertainment study and review of management recommendations. Rheumatol Int 2016;36:1319–1326
3. Cheung WY, Luk KD. Clinical and radiological outcomes after conservative treatment of TB spondylitis: is the 15 years' follow-up in the MRC study long enough? Eur Spine J 2013;22(Suppl 4):594–602 Review
4. Mylona E, Samarkos M, Kakalou E, Fanourgiakis P, Skoutelis A. Pyogenic vertebral osteomyelitis: a systematic review of clinical characteristics. Semin Arthritis Rheum 2009;39:10–17
5. Govender S. Spinal infections. J Bone Joint Surg Br 2005;87:1454–1458

6. Carragee EJ. Pyogenic vertebral osteomyelitis. J Bone Joint Surg Am 1997;79:874–880

7. Geck MJ, Eismont FJ. Pyogenic and fungal lumbar spine infection. In: Herkowitz HN, Dvořák J, Bell GR, Nordin M, Grob D, eds. The Lumbar Spine, 3rd ed. Hagerstown, MD: Lippincott Williams & Wilkins; 2004

8. Akiyama T, Chikuda H, Yasunaga H, Horiguchi H, Fushimi K, Saita K. Incidence and risk factors for mortality of vertebral osteomyelitis: a retrospective analysis using the Japanese diagnosis procedure combination database. BMJ Open 2013;3:e002412

9. Nagashima H, Nanjo Y, Tanida A, Dokai T, Teshima R. Clinical features of spinal infection in individuals older than eighty years. Int Orthop 2012;36:1229–1234

10. Kehrer M, Pedersen C, Jensen TG, Lassen AT. Increasing incidence of pyogenic spondylodiscitis: a 14-year population-based study. J Infect 2014;68:313–320

11. Hutchinson C, Hanger C, Wilkinson T, Sainsbury R, Pithie A. Spontaneous spinal infections in older people. Intern Med J 2009;39:845–848

12. Imajo Y, Taguchi T, Neo M, et al. Complications of spinal surgery for elderly patients with lumbar spinal stenosis in a super-aging country: an analysis of 8033 patients. J Orthop Sci 2017;22:10–15

13. Yamato Y, Matsuyama Y, Hasegawa K, et al; Committee for Adult Deformity, Japanese Scoliosis Society. A Japanese nationwide multicenter survey on perioperative complications of corrective fusion for elderly patients with adult spinal deformity. J Orthop Sci 2017;22:237–242

14. Bernstein DN, Thirukumaran C, Saleh A, Molinari RW, Mesfin A. Complications and readmission after cervical spine surgery in elderly patients: an analysis of 1786 patients. World Neurosurg 2017;103:859–868.e8

15. Rajpal S, Lee Nelson E, Villavicencio AT, et al. Medical complications and mortality in octogenarians undergoing elective spinal fusion surgeries. Acta Neurochir (Wien) 2018;160:171–179

16. Wiley AM, Trueta J. The vascular anatomy of the spine and its relationship to pyogenic vertebral osteomyelitis. J Bone Joint Surg Br 1959;41-B:796–809

17. Nathoo N, Caris EC, Wiener JA, Mendel E. History of the vertebral venous plexus and the significant contributions of Breschet and Batson. Neurosurgery 2011; 69:1007–1014, discussion 1014

18. Tay BK, Deckey J, Hu SS. Spinal infections. J Am Acad Orthop Surg 2002;10:188–197 Review

19. Osti OL, Fraser RD, Vernon-Roberts B. Discitis after discography. The role of prophylactic antibiotics. J Bone Joint Surg Br 1990;72:271–274

20. Falagas ME, Bliziotis IA, Mavrogenis AF, Papagelopoulos PJ. Spondylodiscitis after facet joint steroid injection: a case report and review of the literature. Scand J Infect Dis 2006;38:295–299

21. Sapico FL. Microbiology and antimicrobial therapy of spinal infections. Orthop Clin North Am 1996;27:9–13

22. Yee DK, Samartzis D, Wong YW, Luk KD, Cheung KM. Infective spondylitis in Southern Chinese: a descriptive and comparative study of ninety-one cases. Spine (Phila Pa 1976) 2010;35:635–641

23. Sobottke R, Röllinghoff M, Zarghooni K, et al. Spondylodiscitis in the elderly patient: clinical mid-term results and quality of life. Arch Orthop Trauma Surg 2010;130:1083–1091

24. Belzunegui J, Intxausti JJ, De Dios JR, et al. Haematogenous vertebral osteomyelitis in the elderly. Clin Rheumatol 2000;19:344–347

25. Butler JS, Shelly MJ, Timlin M, Powderly WG, O'Byrne JM. Nontuberculous pyogenic spinal infection in adults: a 12-year experience from a tertiary referral center. Spine 2006;31:2695–2700

26. Eismont FJ, Bohlman HH, Soni PL, Goldberg VM, Freehafer AA. Pyogenic and fungal vertebral osteomyelitis with paralysis. J Bone Joint Surg Am 1983;65:19–29

27. Yee DK, Samartzis D, Wong YW, Luk KD, Cheung KM. Infective spondylitis in Southern Chinese: a descriptive and comparative study of ninety-one cases. Spine 2010;35:635–641

28. Jeong DK, Lee HW, Kwon YM. Clinical value of procalcitonin in patients with spinal infection. J Korean Neurosurg Soc 2015;58:271–275

29. Yoon YK, Jo YM, Kwon HH, et al. Differential diagnosis between tuberculous spondylodiscitis and pyogenic spontaneous spondylodiscitis: a multicenter descriptive and comparative study. Spine J 2015;15:1764–1771

30. An HS, Seldomridge JA. Spinal infections: diagnostic tests and imaging studies. Clin Orthop Relat Res 2006;444:27–33

31. Zhang YH, Zhao CQ, Jiang LS, Chen XD, Dai LY. Modic changes: a systematic review of the literature. Eur Spine J 2008;17:1289–1299

32. Albert HB, Manniche C, Sorensen JS, Deleuran BW. Antibiotic treatment in patients with low-back pain associated with Modic changes type 1 (bone oedema): a pilot study. Br J Sports Med 2008;42:969–973

33. Ohtori S, Koshi T, Yamashita M, et al. Existence of pyogenic spondylitis in Modic type 1 change without other signs of infection: 2-year follow-up. Eur Spine J 2010;19:1200–1205

34. Stumpe KD, Zanetti M, Weishaupt D, Hodler J, Boos N, Von Schulthess GK. FDG positron emission tomography for differentiation of degenerative and infectious endplate abnormalities in the lumbar spine detected on MR imaging. AJR Am J Roentgenol 2002; 179:1151–1157

35. Eguchi Y, Ohtori S, Yamashita M, et al. Diffusion magnetic resonance imaging to differentiate degenerative from infectious endplate abnormalities in the lumbar spine. Spine 2011;36:E198–E202

36. Prodromou ML, Ziakas PD, Poulou LS, Karsaliakos P, Thanos L, Mylonakis E. FDG PET is a robust tool for the diagnosis of spondylodiscitis: a meta-analysis of diagnostic data. Clin Nucl Med 2014;39:330–335

37. Sudhakar P, Sharma AR, Bhushan SM, Ranadhir G, Narsimuhulu G, Rao VV. Efficacy of SPECT over planar bone scan in the diagnosis of solitary vertebral lesions in patients with low back pain. Indian J Nucl Med 2010;25:44–48

38. Bernard L, Dinh A, Ghout I, et al; Duration of Treatment for Spondylodiscitis (DTS) study group. Antibiotic treatment for 6 weeks versus 12 weeks in patients with pyogenic vertebral osteomyelitis: an open-label, non-inferiority, randomised, controlled trial. Lancet 2015;385:875–882

39. Liljenqvist U, Lerner T, Bullmann V, Hackenberg L, Halm H, Winkelmann W. Titanium cages in the surgical treatment of severe vertebral osteomyelitis. Eur Spine J 2003;12:606–612

40. Hee HT, Majd ME, Holt RT, Pienkowski D. Better treatment of vertebral osteomyelitis using posterior stabilization and titanium mesh cages. J Spinal Disord Tech 2002;15:149–156, discussion 156

41. Shetty AP, Viswanathan VK, Kanna RM, Shanmuganathan R. Tubercular spondylodiscitis in elderly is a more severe disease: a report of 66 consecutive patients. Eur Spine J 2017;26:3178–3186

18

Spinal Infections and Pseudarthrosis

Yazeed Gussous, Daniel Beckerman, Nikhil Jain, and Sigurd Berven

Introduction

Infection after spine surgery is a clinically important problem and may be associated with long-term compromise of outcome and pseudarthrosis. The incidence of postoperative infection after spinal surgery is reported to vary between 0.7% and 20%.[1–3] Early infection commonly presents with overt symptoms within 2 to 3 weeks after surgery. Prompt identification and aggressive treatment usually results in resolution of the infection with retention of hardware, without significant long-term sequelae.[1,3–8] Delayed infection, on the other hand, can present months to years after surgery with such constitutional symptoms as chronic pain, wound drainage, implant failure, and pseudarthrosis.[6–11] The Centers for Disease Control and Prevention (CDC) proposed a duration of 1 year as the standard time period for a delayed deep infection after surgery if an implant is present.[12] Reported rates of pseudarthrosis following surgical site infection (SSI) range from 5 to 20%.[9,13] Overall, the incidence of pseudarthrosis after lumbar fusion is estimated to be 5 to 35%, and in up to 50% of cases after cervical fusion.[14,15] Patients usually present with recurrent pain or neurologic symptoms, and pseudarthrosis is responsible for up to half of the revision surgeries. Whereas 30% patients may be asymptomatic, the symptoms of pseudarthrosis are nonspecific and can be due to underlying infection, disease progression, implant failure, or adjacent segment disease.[14,15] Therefore, symptomatic pseudarthrosis should be investigated by a complete clinical, radiological, and laboratory workup to rule out underlying infection as a possible secondary cause.[3,14–16]

A high index of suspicion for subclinical infection should be maintained in the absence of clear signs of infection, as a recent report found positive intraoperative cultures in up to 44% cases of revisions for pseudarthrosis, which were otherwise not suspected of harboring infection.[16] These findings indicate that the likelihood of infection in cases of pseudarthrosis of the spine is high, and infection should be considered in the differential diagnosis of acute and delayed pseudarthrosis and implant failure. The surgical treatment of infection in the presence of a solid fusion is generally agreed to consist of debridement and removal of instrumentation.[1,3,5–11,13,17,18] Infection in the setting of an incomplete fusion is an important and common clinical challenge, and strategies for management may include primary or delayed implant exchange. The purpose of this chapter is to describe the pathophysiology of postoperative infection and pseudarthrosis in spine surgery and to present an evidence-based approach to the management of postoperative spine infection and pseudarthrosis.

The Problem of Biofilm

Bacteria can adhere to the surface of foreign materials and form a matrix of extracellular polymeric substances, within which they embed.[3,10] These foreign materials include devascularized autograft, allograft, and hardware, which are commonly used in spinal fusion.[19] This biofilm offers protection against antibiotics, phagocytes, and other immune responses. These bacteria often demonstrate an altered phenotype with respect to their growth rate and gene expression. All these factors lead to increased difficulty in isolating and eradicating the microorganisms responsible for infection. Most of the common organisms that cause postoperative spinal infections, such as *Staphylococcus* and *Propionibacterium,* have the ability to produce biofilm.[3] The implant material has also been shown to affect the rate of bacterial adherence and subsequent biofilm production. Studies have found that pure titanium has a lower infection rate as compared with titanium alloys and stainless steel.[20,21] Interbody cages made of polyetheretherketone (PEEK) are widely used for cervical and lumbar fusion, but show a relatively high risk of biofilm formation.[22,23] Silicon nitride, a relatively recent entrant in the United States market, unlike titanium and PEEK, has a positively charged hydrophilic surface and has been shown to inhibit bacterial colonization and biofilm formation.[22,23] Surgeon familiarity with materials and the propensity of bacterial adherence is important when considering the use of hardware in the presence of infection.

The age of the biofilm is also important as early infections have less tenacious and immature biofilm, leading to adequate removal by debridement and antibiotics.[3] Maturation of biofilm and persistence of infection without implant removal is an important consideration in the management of delayed infection,[1,3] especially in the presence of unhealed fusion. Culturing microorganisms from mature biofilm colonies on implants is difficult and, even if grown, antibiotic susceptibility testing is often inaccurate.[3,11] *Propionibacterium* is a facultative anaerobe implicated in a significant number of late infections, and requires prolonged culture for detection.[3,7,16,18] Sampredo et al[24] described a technique of vortexing and sonication of spinal implants preceding culture, and was shown to be more sensitive than peri-implant cultures.

Diagnosis

Clinically the recurrence or persistence of pain after fusion should lead to a high suspicion for the presence of pseudarthrosis. Radiographically, evidence of subsidence, hardware failure, or implant loosening suggests pseudarthrosis. The time at which pseudarthrosis is considered established is not uniform, and is not described after spinal fusion. Based on the trauma literature for fractures, it is considered that failure to show any progressive radiographic evidence of fusion for at least 3 months after the time period in which normal fracture union (usually 3 to 6 months) would have occurred, is evidence of nonunion.[25] If present, constitutional symptoms, pain at incision site, tenderness to palpation, or wound drainage indicates an underlying infection.[3]

The initial assessment of pseudarthrosis should include plain radiographs with flexion-extension views and thin-cut computed tomography (CT).[14,15] In addition to these modalities, the workup for infection should include laboratory markers such as total leukocyte count (TLC), erythrocyte sedimentation rate (ESR), and C-reactive protein (CRP). CRP has been shown to be more sensitive for the detection of infection as it is relatively stable for each individual, has a narrow normal range, and is minimally affected by medications and other pathologies (except liver failure).[2,3,7]

Given the low virulence of microorganisms causing delayed infection, clinical signs and elevated laboratory markers may be absent. Therefore, a degree of suspicion is warranted in all cases of pseudarthrosis.[16,18] Measurement of nutritional parameters, including serum albumin, total protein, calcium, and vitamin D is important to identify opportunity to optimize immune function and bone healing capacity.

Magnetic resonance imaging (MRI) with and without contrast is of great value for diagnosing diskitis, osteomyelitis, and epidural abscess,[3,8] although the presence of instrumentation requires special protocols for metal artifact suppression.[8] Additional modalities that may be considered include radionuclide bone scintigraphy using technetium-99m methylene diphosphonate (MDP), especially in cases of inconclusive MRI findings.[26] Whereas technetium-99m MDP scan may be affected by underlying bone formation, gallium-67– and indium-111–labeled leukocyte scans are more specific for infection.[3] ^{18}F-fluorodeoxyglucose (FDG)–positron emission tomography (PET) can be a useful modality for diagnosing delayed infection, but is expensive and requires equipment that is not universally available.[27] Even in the presence of unequivocal clinical, laboratory, and imaging findings of infection, definitive diagnosis can only be reached by bacteriological examination of infected tissues.[26] Biopsy is considered superior to blood cultures in pathogen detection and can be routinely performed in suspicious cases. Although user dependent, CT-guided biopsy is a useful technique to obtain microbiological diagnosis and antibiotic suseptibility.[26,28]

Shifflett et al[16] evaluated 578 cases of "presumed aseptic" revision spine surgeries at a single institution between 2008 and 2013. In their analysis, they included patients who had a negative clinical, laboratory, and radiographic workup for infection and hence "presumed aseptic." They had obtained an average of 5.5 intraoperative cultures (range, 1–14) in 19.4% ($n = 112$) of cases based on the surgeon's intraoperative clinical judgement or as routine. Of all the cases that had positive intraoperative cultures ($n = 45$), pseudarthrosis was the primary revision diagnosis in 53.3% patients. Interestingly, 55.6% of all uninstrumented cases had a positive culture as opposed to only 32.9% of the instrumented cases. In patients revised for pseudarthrosis, *Propionibacterium acnes* was cultured in 54.2% cases, *Staphylococcus* species in 58.3%, polymicrobial infections

in 25%, and gram-negative organisms in 12.5% cases. *P. acnes* is a common culprit in delayed infection and has been implicated in cases of pseudarthrosis.[3,7–9,16,18] Additionally, given the association between *P. acnes* and degenerative disk disease, the authors hypothesized that this exposure at the index surgery could very well play a role in the subsequent development of pseudarthrosis. The limitations of this retrospective study precluded the formulation of any specific recommendations, but the authors emphasized that applying clinical judgment and determining the presence of pseudarthrosis warrant a high degree of suspicion in the absence of clear indicators of infection.

Management

There is a consensus in the literature on postoperative spinal infection that early infection is best managed by debridement, hardware retention, and systemic antibiotic therapy.[1,3–8] The rationale behind hardware retention is to allow time for union to occur and to minimize the risk of instability and neurologic deficit. The majority of recommendations on the management of delayed infection are applied after solid fusion occurs, in which case debridement and hardware removal is indicated.[1,3,5–11,13,17,18] In situation where there is a highly virulent or drug-resistant pathogen, early removal of hardware in conjunction with antibiotic treatment should be considered, along with activity modification and bracing followed by delayed reimplantation. Pseudarthrosis secondary to infection, however, usually presents late, and the evidence on the management of established pseudarthrosis in the presence of infection is unclear.

Hedequist et al[17] presented their experience with 1,771 patients who underwent an instrumented spine fusion for scoliosis, kyphosis, or spondylolisthesis. In their series, delayed infections persisted when hardware was left in place. Further debridement was necessary, and only hardware removal led to healing of the wound. They found that adequate debridement is not possible with the hardware in place as the spaces underneath rods and anchor spots are inaccessible. Second, immediate replacement of hardware would be futile given the colonized bed. Finally, repeat debridements and prolonged hospital stays significantly increase the health care costs. Although the authors did not have any patient presenting with an unstable spine or nonunion, they suggested that these patients may need retention of hardware until union occurs.

There is evidence, mostly from the scoliosis literature, that even in the presence of radiographic evidence of fusion, removal of the hardware can lead to a loss of correction and pseudarthrosis.[1,3,17] Clark and Shufflebarger[11] reported on 1,247 scoliosis surgeries, and suggested that removal of all metallic hardware is necessary for resolution of late infection. However, if a pseudarthrosis is present and is symptomatic after implant removal, then re-instrumentation with titanium implants can be done. Steel implants are known to form metallic debris from corrosion and fretting, which constitutes an environment for incubation of dormant or low-virulent organisms.[3,11] The use of titanium precludes the possibility of nickel and chromium sensitivity that can cause sterile inflammation and an increased risk of infection. Titanium also has a low risk of biofilm formation.[11,20,21]

Cahill et al[29] did a retrospective review of 1,543 patients who underwent surgery for pediatric spinal deformity. Their reported incidence of pseudarthrosis and infection was 25% ($n = 13/51$). These patients required an average of 1.2 procedures to treat the pseudarthrosis; treatment was successful in only six patients. All patients had a significant progression of deformity on follow-up, which was independent of whether or not the pseudarthrosis healed. The authors re-instrumented the spines that had an inadequate fusion mass, but their report did not specify the procedures used or the outcomes in these patients.

Rihn et al[30] retrospectively studied 236 patients treated for idiopathic scoliosis. They reported that none of the patients diagnosed with pseudarthrosis at the time of debridement underwent re-instrumentation surgery after clearance of the infection. These patients

did develop progression of the spine curve, but their outcome scores were similar to those of patients who did not have infection. They argued against the need for revision surgery after infection and hardware removal, even if pseudarthrosis or curve progression is present. Previous studies have also supported the fact that the amount of radiographic curve correction and fusion success are not always correlated with patient-reported outcomes.[31,32] Mirovsky et al[32] successfully treated deep infections and found improved clinical outcomes despite suboptimal fusion rates. These findings suggest important considerations when contemplating aggressive treatment of pseudarthrosis.

In the absence of clear guidelines, hardware reinsertion should be based on the surgeon's intraoperative clinical judgment. The condition of the operative bed and the adequacy of the debridement should determine if immediate reimplantation should be done. If there is frank purulence covering the instrumentation, then it is better to wait at least 1 week before planning reimplantation and administer antibiotics in the meantime. However, if the wound has mainly fibrinous material that is easily debrided to obtain vascular and healthy tissue, then reinserting new hardware at the same time could be considered.[12]

Falavigna et al,[4] in their review, supported the retention of instrumentation and implants to achieve the primary goals of surgery. They postulated that stability provided by instrumentation decreases micro-motion and inflammation, and promotes bone healing. Ha and Kim[33] hypothesized that implants may be safely left in situ to provide stability for fusion. However, in their case series of infected posterior lumbar interbody fusions (PLIFs), they were unsuccessful in clearing infection even after serial wound debridement and irrigation. They chose to treat these infections more aggressively and opted for wide anterior debridement, implant removal, and anterior interbody fusion with autogenous bone graft. They reported good fusion and clinical outcomes in these patients. The posterior removal of cages was considered a highly complicated procedure due to postoperative and postinfection scarring.

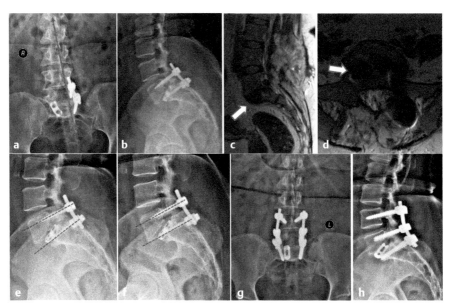

Fig. 18.1 This 54-year-old woman had been initially treated for L5-S1 lytic spondylolisthesis with a transforaminal lumbar interbody fusion (TLIF). However, because she developed radiculopathy on the right side with wound infection postoperatively, the surgeon had removed the right L5 and S1 screws and treated her with antibiotics. She was relatively pain free for 2 years, and when she presented to us in the third year, she had significant back pain and right-side radiculopathy. **(a)** Radiographs showed a sciatic list and **(b)** loss of lordosis. **(c,d)** Magnetic resonance imaging (MRI) showed subchondral edema in the S1 vertebra, indicative of subclinical infection *(arrow)*. **(e,f)** Stress radiographs showed movement at the L5-S1 level, suggestive of pseudarthrosis. **(g,h)** The patient was treated with implant removal and extension of instrumentation, with interbody debridement and fusion at L5-S1 and an instrumented posterolateral fusion at L4–L5.

The question of whether metal hardware can be used for reconstruction in the presence of infection has been addressed by several studies.[11,34–39] Shetty et al[37] successfully treated 27 cases of pyogenic spondylodiskitis with transforaminal lumbar interbody fusion (TLIF). They did not have any instances of cage migration, loosening, or infection recurrence with a minimum 2-year follow-up. They concluded that TLIF with titanium cages may be safely used for treating pyogenic lumbar spondylodiskitis provided that thorough debridement is achieved, appropriate antibiotic coverage is started, and close follow-up is possible. An et al[38] and Lee and Suh[39] hypothesized that the high vascularity of cancellous bone in the vertebral body coupled with thorough debridement and antibiotics facilitates the placement of metal hardware, including interbody spacers, with a low risk of infection recurrence and biofilm formation (**Fig. 18.1**).

Recommendations on antibiotic therapy vary widely. Whenever available, the choice should be based on the susceptibility results.[3] Richards and Emara[9] recommended 2 to 5 days of intravenous (IV) antibiotics followed by 1 to 2 weeks of oral antibiotics for the treatment of delayed infection after hardware removal, whereas Rihn et al[30] used only IV antibiotics for 6 weeks and reported successful clearance of infection in their seven cases. Clark and Shufflebarger[11] recommended 2 to 3 days of IV antibiotics followed by 10 days of oral therapy. Kowalski et al[6] used a 6-week IV schedule followed by 6 weeks of oral antibiotics to successfully treat patients who had their hardware retained. Collins et al[18] effectively treated infection with an average of mean 4 weeks of IV administration followed by 5 weeks of oral suppressive therapy. There was no relapse in those patients who had their hardware removed, as compared with 40% recurrence in patients with retained hardware. Lifelong suppression may be needed if hardware is retained, and such a decision should be based on the patient's health status, fusion success, and causative organism.[8]

Chapter Summary

Pseudarthrosis may develop as a result of postoperative infection, or delayed infection may develop in the presence of instability or an unhealed fusion. In the presence of nonspecific symptoms of pseudarthrosis, a complete clinical, laboratory, and radiological workup for infection is required. Delayed infections are often low grade, and the possibility of a subclinical infection in the absence of clear signs should always be considered. It should be kept in mind that up to 30% cases of pseudarthrosis may be asymptomatic and hence its mere presence does not warrant treatment. The clearance of infection will usually require debridement, hardware removal, and culture-directed antibiotics. Cultures should be taken meticulously and incubated for prolonged periods to isolate slow-growing pathogens such as *P. acnes*. Extensive surgeries such as those for scoliosis may demand re-instrumentation due to concerns of significant loss of correction or nonunion. Re-instrumentation with titanium can be done as a single stage or at a later date depending on the infection load, the adequacy of the debridement, and the patient's suitability for anesthesia. Interbody fusions may be revised with titanium cages with auto- or al-

lograft after adequate debridement and removal of all infected hardware either in the same setting or in a staged manner. Revision fusion may be approached by a route other than primary surgery to avoid scarred tissue planes. Reconstruction strategies to tackle pseudarthrosis and achieve fusion can be pursued effectively with aggressive debridement, reinstrumentation to gain spine stability, antibiotics, and wound coverage techniques.

Pearls

◆ Consider the diagnosis of infection whenever a patient presents with pseudarthrosis, and consider the diagnosis of pseudarthrosis whenever a patient presents with infection.
◆ Consider ordering preoperative and intraoperative biopsies and cultures when working up a patient with pseudarthrosis.
◆ Eradication of delayed infection is more likely after the removal of the hardware, given the presence of biofilm, and complete debridement may not be possible over and around the hardware.
◆ The explanted hardware and debrided tissue should be cultured meticulously for an adequate time period to isolate slow-growing and fastidious pathogens.
◆ Elimination of infection alone may achieve good patient outcomes, and the need to address pseudarthrosis should be made on a case-by-case basis.

Pitfalls

◆ Pseudarthrosis alone may be asymptomatic in up to a third of patients.
◆ In all cases of symptomatic pseudarthrosis, make sure to rule out infection, implant failure, disease progression, and adjacent segment disease.
◆ Ask the microbiology laboratory to maintain cultures for 14 days to enable identification of slow-growing pathogens causing delayed infections.
◆ Retention of hardware to allow healing of fusion in the presence of infection often results in repeated debridements, prolonged administration of antibiotics, additional patient morbidity, and higher health care costs.
◆ Re-instrumentation of the spine to prevent loss of radiographic curve correction and to achieve successful fusion may not always result in successful patient-reported outcomes.

References
Five Must-Read References

1. Lall RR, Wong AP, Lall RR, Lawton CD, Smith ZA, Dahdaleh NS. Evidence-based management of deep wound infection after spinal instrumentation. J Clin Neurosci 2015;22:238–242

2. Radcliff KE, Neusner AD, Millhouse PW, et al. What is new in the diagnosis and prevention of spine surgical site infections. Spine J 2015;15:336–347

3. Kasliwal MK, Tan LA, Traynelis VC. Infection with spinal instrumentation: review of pathogenesis, diagnosis, prevention, and management. Surg Neurol Int 2013;4(Suppl 5):S392–S403

4. Falavigna A, Righesso Neto O, Fonseca GP, Nervo M. [Management of deep wound infections in spinal lumbar fusions]. Arq Neuropsiquiatr 2006;64:1001–1004

5. Mok JM, Guillaume TJ, Talu U, et al. Clinical outcome of deep wound infection after instrumented posterior spinal fusion: a matched cohort analysis. Spine 2009;34:578–583

6. Kowalski TJ, Berbari EF, Huddleston PM, Steckelberg JM, Mandrekar JN, Osmon DR. The management and outcome of spinal implant infections: contemporary retrospective cohort study. Clin Infect Dis 2007;44:913–920

7. Gerometta A, Rodriguez Olaverri JC, Bitan F. Infections in spinal instrumentation. Int Orthop 2012;36:457–464

8. Hegde V, Meredith DS, Kepler CK, Huang RC. Management of postoperative spinal infections. World J Orthop 2012;3:182–189

9. Richards BR, Emara KM. Delayed infections after posterior TSRH spinal instrumentation for idiopathic scoliosis: revisited. Spine 2001;26:1990–1996

10. Bose B. Delayed infection after instrumented spine surgery: case reports and review of the literature. Spine J 2003;3:394–399

11. Clark CE, Shufflebarger HL. Late-developing infection in instrumented idiopathic scoliosis. Spine 1999;24:1909–1912

12. Maruo K, Berven SH. Outcome and treatment of postoperative spine surgical site infections: predictors of treatment success and failure. J Orthop Sci 2014;19:398–404

13. Weinstein MA, McCabe JP, Cammisa FP Jr. Postoperative spinal wound infection: a review of 2,391 consecutive index procedures. J Spinal Disord 2000;13:422–426

14. Leven D, Cho SK. Pseudarthrosis of the cervical spine: risk factors, diagnosis and management. Asian Spine J 2016;10:776–786

15. Chun DS, Baker KC, Hsu WK. Lumbar pseudarthrosis: a review of current diagnosis and treatment. Neurosurg Focus 2015;39:E10

16. Shifflett GD, Bjerke-Kroll BT, Nwachukwu BU, et al. Microbiologic profile of infections in presumed aseptic revision spine surgery. Eur Spine J 2016;25:3902–3907

17. Hedequist D, Haugen A, Hresko T, Emans J. Failure of attempted implant retention in spinal deformity delayed surgical site infections. Spine 2009;34:60–64

18. Collins I, Wilson-MacDonald J, Chami G, et al. The diagnosis and management of infection following instrumented spinal fusion. Eur Spine J 2008;17:445–450

19. DE LA Garza-Ramos R, Bydon M, Macki M, et al. Instrumented fusion in the setting of primary spinal infection. J Neurosurg Sci 2017;61:64–76

20. Schildhauer TA, Robie B, Muhr G, Köller M. Bacterial adherence to tantalum versus commonly used orthopedic metallic implant materials. J Orthop Trauma 2006;20:476–484

21. Soultanis KC, Pyrovolou N, Zahos KA, et al. Late postoperative infection following spinal instrumentation: stainless steel versus titanium implants. J Surg Orthop Adv 2008;17:193–199

22. Webster TJ, Patel AA, Rahaman MN, Sonny Bal B. Anti-infective and osteointegration properties of silicon nitride, poly(ether ether ketone), and titanium implants. Acta Biomater 2012;8:4447–4454 Erratum in: Acta Biomater 2014;10:1485–1486

23. Gorth DJ, Puckett S, Ercan B, Webster TJ, Rahaman M, Bal BS. Decreased bacteria activity on Si_3N_4 surfaces compared with PEEK or titanium. Int J Nanomedicine 2012;7:4829–4840

24. Sampedro MF, Huddleston PM, Piper KE, et al. A biofilm approach to detect bacteria on removed spinal implants. Spine 2010;35:1218–1224

25. Heppenstall RB. Fracture Treatment and Healing. Philadelphia: WB Saunders; 1980

26. Duarte RM, Vaccaro AR. Spinal infection: state of the art and management algorithm. Eur Spine J 2013;22:2787–2799

27. Strobel K, Stumpe KD. PET/CT in musculoskeletal infection. Semin Musculoskelet Radiol 2007;11:353–364

28. de Lucas EM, González Mandly A, Gutiérrez A, et al. CT-guided fine-needle aspiration in vertebral osteomyelitis: true usefulness of a common practice. Clin Rheumatol 2009;28:315–320

29. Cahill PJ, Warnick DE, Lee MJ, et al. Infection after spinal fusion for pediatric spinal deformity: thirty years of experience at a single institution. Spine 2010;35:1211–1217

30. Rihn JA, Lee JY, Ward WT. Infection after the surgical treatment of adolescent idiopathic scoliosis: evalua-

tion of the diagnosis, treatment, and impact on clinical outcomes. Spine 2008;33:289–294

31. Wilson PL, Newton PO, Wenger DR, et al. A multicenter study analyzing the relationship of a standardized radiographic scoring system of adolescent idiopathic scoliosis and the Scoliosis Research Society outcomes instrument. Spine 2002;27:2036–2040

32. Mirovsky Y, Floman Y, Smorgick Y, et al. Management of deep wound infection after posterior lumbar interbody fusion with cages. J Spinal Disord Tech 2007; 20:127–131

33. Ha KY, Kim YH. Postoperative spondylitis after posterior lumbar interbody fusion using cages. Eur Spine J 2004;13:419–424

34. Rayes M, Colen CB, Bahgat DA, et al. Safety of instrumentation in patients with spinal infection. J Neurosurg Spine 2010;12:647–659

35. Kuklo TR, Potter BK, Bell RS, Moquin RR, Rosner MK. Single-stage treatment of pyogenic spinal infection with titanium mesh cages. J Spinal Disord Tech 2006; 19:376–382

36. Sundararaj GD, Amritanand R, Venkatesh K, Arockiaraj J. The use of titanium mesh cages in the reconstruction of anterior column defects in active spinal infections: can we rest the crest? Asian Spine J 2011; 5:155–161

37. Shetty AP, Aiyer SN, Kanna RM, Maheswaran A, Rajasekaran S. Pyogenic lumbar spondylodiscitis treated with transforaminal lumbar interbody fusion: safety and outcomes. Int Orthop 2016;40:1163–1170

38. An KC, Kim JY, Kim TH, et al. Posterior lumbar interbody fusion using compressive bone graft with allograft and autograft in the pyogenic discitis. Asian Spine J 2012;6:15–21

39. Lee JS, Suh KT. Posterior lumbar interbody fusion with an autogenous iliac crest bone graft in the treatment of pyogenic spondylodiscitis. J Bone Joint Surg Br 2006;88:765–770

Index